HOW
NOT TO
GET SICK

Also by Benjamin Bikman, PhD

*Why We Get Sick: The Hidden Epidemic at the Root of
Most Chronic Disease—and How to Fight It*

Also by Diana Keuilian

*The Recipe Hacker: Comfort Foods Without Soy,
Dairy, Cane Sugar, Gluten, and Grain*

*The Recipe Hacker Confidential: Break the
Code to Cooking Mouthwatering & Good-For-You Meals
Without Grains, Gluten, Dairy, Soy, or Cane Sugar*

*Always Eat After 7 PM: The Revolutionary Rule-Breaking
Diet That Lets You Enjoy Huge Dinners, Desserts, and Indulgent
Snacks—While Burning Fat Overnight* (by Joel Marion,
with recipes by Diana Keuilian)

HOW NOT TO GET SICK

A COOKBOOK AND GUIDE
to Prevent and Reverse Insulin Resistance,
Lose Weight, and Fight Chronic Disease

**Benjamin Bikman, PhD
and Diana Keuilian**

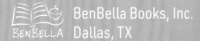 BenBella Books, Inc.
Dallas, TX

How Not to Get Sick copyright © 2024 by Benjamin Bikman and Diana Keuilian
Food photography by Diana Keuilian
Exercise photography by Breezy Ann Photography/Anna Frenkel

BENBELLA

BenBella Books, Inc.
10440 N. Central Expressway
Suite 800
Dallas, TX 75231
benbellabooks.com
Send feedback to feedback@benbellabooks.com
BenBella is a federally registered trademark.

Printed in China
10 9 8 7 6 5 4 3 2 1

Library of Congress Control Number: 2023039788
ISBN 978-1-63774-454-3 (trade paperback)
ISBN 978-1-63774-455-0 (electronic)

Editing by Claire Schulz
Copyediting by Karen Wise
Proofreading by Sarah Vostok and Lisa Story
Indexing by WordCo Indexing Services, Inc.
Text design by Paul Nielson, Faceout Studio
Text composition by Aaron Edmiston
Cover design by Brigid Pearson
Printed by KS Printing

Special discounts for bulk sales are available. Please contact bulkorders@benbellabooks.com.

For our families

and

For the courageous reader willing to take
the journey to improve their health.

CONTENTS

Introduction

As a metabolic scientist, one of the most frustrating parts of my job is the expectation of how we share evidence: we conduct experiments, analyze the results, then share what we find in a peer-reviewed publication.

Even if that information is usable and helpful, very few people ever read these science publications, and the information is generally not conveyed to the public in an actionable way.

In 2017, I was pushing against these trends. I thought, "If I have relevant answers to important questions, I should find a way to translate these answers into practical solutions to real-world problems." (This thought was largely responsible for me starting to write my first book, *Why We Get Sick*.) At the same time, I wanted to test some of my ideas on people struggling with their metabolic health. To do this, I recruited a local clinic for help.

The clinical team and I identified 11 middle-aged women who were recently diagnosed with type 2 diabetes, which is a consequence of insulin resistance. The patients were offered a choice of either a prescription for an antidiabetic drug or a "prescription" for better nutrition. All 11 elected to follow the nutrition counsel. By following simple rules (the same used in this book), without ever taking any medication, they went on to improve their insulin resistance to such a degree that they had *no evidence of diabetes*—they had reversed their poor metabolic health.[1] This strategy worked expressly because we emphasized the role of insulin.

If you haven't read my first book, when you see the word *insulin*, you may think that any problem with insulin is only a problem for people with diabetes.

Even as a scientist, I used to think that too. Then came my moment of enlightenment. During my postdoctoral fellowship in metabolic disorders, I stumbled on a scientific article titled "Alzheimer's Disease Is Type 3 Diabetes,"[2] which outlined the myriad connections between insulin resistance and deficits in memory and learning. Soon after, I was searching through the breadth of biomedical literature to find other connections between chronic disorders and insulin resistance. What I found was enough to fill a book (and, well, I did)—insulin resistance was an essential part of almost every chronic health disorder. High blood pressure? It's likely insulin resistance.[3] Ringing in the ears? Could be insulin resistance.[4] Infertility? Probably insulin resistance.[5] The list goes on.

Before going further, let's make sure we have a common understanding of insulin resistance. I often describe it as a coin with two sides. On one side, there is the altered insulin effect at some cells of the body, or *reduced insulin action*. This is the pure form of insulin resistance—some cells are literally resistant to what insulin is trying to tell them to do. The other side of the coin is *hyperinsulinemia*—chronically elevated blood insulin levels. A point of emphasis: these always come together. Remember, the altered insulin effect and the elevated blood insulin are two sides of the *same coin*. In other words, there is no reduced insulin action without elevated blood insulin. To fully understand how insulin resistance contributes to so many disorders, we need to keep the two sides of the coin in mind; in specific instances, one side can be more relevant than the other. For example, Alzheimer's disease arises partly because insulin isn't working well in certain brain regions; this results in the brain not being able to get enough energy from blood glucose. However, in polycystic ovary syndrome (PCOS; the most common cause of female infertility), the ovary cells are as responsive to insulin as they ever were; the problem arises due to the excess insulin stimulating the ovary cells too much and disrupting sex hormone production.

The two-pillared definition of insulin resistance is deliberately reflected in the two-pronged approach outlined in this book. In order to fully prevent or

> You may think that any problem with insulin is only a problem for people with diabetes. Even as a scientist, I used to think that too. Then came my moment of enlightenment.

reverse insulin resistance, we need to both improve the compromised insulin action on cells *and* reduce the chronically elevated insulin levels. The first of these—helping insulin work better—is very effectively addressed with physical activity. By moving the body, in all kinds of ways, we stimulate our muscles to pull in glucose much more readily. This helps lower blood glucose levels to fasting levels and, as a result, helps insulin come down. Similarly, yet distinctly, by changing what and when we eat, we can help our blood insulin levels come down and stay down. This strategy helps resolve the second aspect of insulin resistance.

Understanding insulin resistance—what it is, where it comes from, and what to do about it—was the focus of *Why We Get Sick*; it was a book I *had* to write to help create a conversation about insulin resistance that just wasn't happening. However, as much as I wanted to include a section in that book on how to fight insulin resistance, I feared I wouldn't be able to say it all or say it well. After reading *Why We Get Sick*, you might have had a moment when you thought, "What now?" Well, here you are.

I'm a scientist and professor—my strengths are understanding problems and being able to teach these to others. I'm not a very good life coach. Laying out the actual action plan requires experience that goes beyond the laboratory. That's where Diana comes in. In a way, this is two books in one—the first part is the classroom, and the second and third parts are what happens in your home. Where I can teach you the relevance and scope of the problem, Diana can teach you what to do about it. I have the map, if you will, and can draw the line from point of origin to the destination, but Diana is the tour guide who actually gets you there. In working together, with Diana fully understanding and appreciating the relevance and origins of insulin resistance, the dietary and exercise plans you'll read about are the perfect practical implementation of the ideas borne from the best scientific evidence.

In this book, Diana and I translate the best available scientific evidence into the best available lifestyle solutions to prevent and reverse insulin resistance. First, we want to start by determining where you are with regard to

> **This book is the road map and your personal virtual tour guide to help you get to better metabolic health.**

insulin resistance (chapter 1). Then, we explore what and when to eat (chapters 2 through 5), along with an overview of nondiet factors (exercise, cold-therapy, etc.; chapters 6 and 7). Following this, we lay out a threefold approach, depending on where you are metabolically speaking. After this, Diana really takes you into the specifics of what the plans should look like, including exercise protocols and carb-conscious recipes.

Wherever you are, this book is the road map and your personal virtual tour guide to help you get to better metabolic health. I wish you all the best on your journey.

Yours in health,

Benjamin Bikman

A note of caution

If you have type 2 diabetes or other insulin resistance-related diseases (hypertension, PCOS, etc.) and you take medications, please discuss all lifestyle changes with your clinical team. Seriously. The lifestyle plans outlined in this book will likely result in such dramatic changes in your level of insulin resistance that you will need to monitor your medication needs to prevent potential harmful problems. For example, blood pressure improves so rapidly in some people that if you're taking a blood pressure medication *while* improving your insulin resistance, your blood pressure could get dangerously low. Again: please discuss your plan with your clinical team so they can monitor your medication needs effectively while you improve your metabolic health without drugs—which is the only way to truly reverse insulin resistance.

A Note from Diana

Hi friend,

When I first read *Why We Get Sick* and got schooled on insulin resistance and metabolic health, I felt like a truth bomb had been set off in front of me, blowing up my understanding (or misunderstanding) of health and fitness. Wading through the rubble of what I thought I knew, disbelief, confusion, frustration, and, yes, even anger ran through me. Why was I just learning about this now after decades of running on the fitness–health–weight loss hamster wheel? Why wasn't this research taught and shared through schools and mainstream media? And, most importantly, what am I going to do with this liberating, life-changing information?

My name is Diana Keuilian, and I'm here to coach you (and coax you) through the practical steps to living an insulin-sensitive lifestyle. I'm not a scientist (don't ask me to pronounce chylomicrons or myokines!), I'm just a regular mom with a background in fitness and a knack for making healthy recipes that taste every bit as delicious as your former (waist-expanding, insulin-spiking) favorites. Most importantly, I've learned to implement Dr. Bikman's research on how to reverse and prevent insulin resistance and actively, joyfully live this truly *healthy lifestyle*.

But what does that actually mean? We've been brainwashed with many a "golden rule" of fitness that has turned out to be a metabolic health myth, including but not limited to:

* Eat low fat. (And make sure it's "healthy" fat, never saturated fats!)

* Avoid foods high in cholesterol, and don't eat too much meat or dairy.
(You better not eat that egg yolk!)

* Eat small meals every couple of hours to burn fat.
(Don't let your metabolism "crash"!)

* Power your workout with carbs.
(Your muscles need fuel!)

* Don't go too long between meals.
(You will lose muscle!)

* Smoothies and fresh juices are super healthy.
(Especially if it's green!)

* Fasting is dangerous and extreme.
(Why would you kill your metabolism like that?)

* All calories are the same.
(And you better count them!)

I've worked for 20+ years in the fitness industry, and despite my experience, expertise, and passion for the subject, I struggled at times to understand what it truly meant to live a healthy lifestyle. So if I have been confused, you can imagine how clients walking into the gym felt (maybe you are one of them!). Being fit and healthy can seem like the ultimate Rubik's Cube: a time-consuming puzzle that very few solve. This confusion is made worse with contradictory information and temporary results. For instance, sure, it's possible to lose fat and gain muscle eating a calorie-controlled, low-fat, high-protein diet and doing long, intense workouts. However, it's not sustainable or efficient. A telltale sign is the overwhelming number of fitness professionals who struggle to maintain their own ideal body weight. I've been there myself many times. Mainstream health and fitness is frustrating, it's confusing, and we are clearly set up for failure. Without an understanding of the impact that insulin has on fat burning, we're basically white-knuckling through health and fitness.

I've since shifted from my grueling conventional fitness plan (low fat, high protein, several meals per day, daily workout regimen) to an insulin-sensitive lifestyle (very low carb, high fat, moderate protein, daily intermittent fasting, occasional extended fasts, and 3 or 4 workouts per week). And the results have spoken for themselves. For the first time ever, I've maintained sculpted abs—without being a slave to my workout routine and without having to think about diet and exercise all day long. As I'll show you in chapter 12, working out doesn't have to take a ton of time or special equipment to give you results. The fasting lifestyle (which Dr. Bikman will tell you about in chapter 2) is incredibly liberating, though it does sound strange and scary at first, especially when you're accustomed to "fueling your metabolism" with snacks and meals all day long. Most snacking and small meals throughout the day are more habit than necessity. I've come to love the feeling of fasting and the sustained, alert energy that it fills me with. And there's no question that food is less of a hassle and less of an expense when fasting for most of the day, and then cooking a satisfying, high-fat, moderate-protein, super-low-carb dinner for the family in the evening. (I also enjoy a weekly higher-carb meal and never restrict myself from enjoying the occasional indulgence.) Once you break the cycle of your current eating style, you'll find freedom that comes along with your shrinking waistline and rising insulin sensitivity.

And who knew that an insulin-sensitive lifestyle could be so enjoyable? As you'll see in chapter 13, with some smart swaps, you can still enjoy all the flavors and textures of the comfort foods you love—like my Mini Pizzas (page 226), BBQ Pulled Pork Sliders (page 176), and Layered Caramel Cookie Bars (page 240). Living carb-conscious doesn't mean you're doomed to a life of Cobb salad on repeat (though I've got a recipe for a really delicious one on page 146, so don't miss it!).

I'll be here to guide and support you along your way to better health. Let's do this!

To your best life,

Diana Keuilian

Diana Keuilian

The Science

Am I Insulin Resistant?

Here's some bad news—you probably have insulin resistance. It's unfortunate, but, statistically, it's very likely the case. A 2019 study surveyed the metabolic health of American adults from 2009 to 2016.[1] The study authors defined "metabolic health" as an individual being in a good range in five metrics: waist circumference, fasting blood glucose, blood pressure, and two blood lipid measurements (triglycerides and high-density lipoprotein cholesterol). The results of their work were startling: *only 12% of adults in the United States were in healthy ranges in all metrics.* So it's likely that you fall into the other group—among the 88% of adults who have an unhealthy level in at least one of those five categories.

You might ask: How has the problem gotten so bad? There are numerous answers to this, but an important one is that most people have an incorrect view of metabolic health, particularly as it pertains to one of the most notorious (and common) metabolic issues, type 2 diabetes.

The conventional clinical view of type 2 diabetes is glucose-centric—patients and their doctors just keep an eye on the blood glucose (sometimes

What Is Insulin?

Insulin is an anabolic hormone, which means it generally promotes the growth of tissues within the body. Because cells need to grow, it's no surprise that every single cell in the body has insulin receptors—little docking stations for insulin. Across all of the diverse cells of the body, insulin generally helps cells grow by activating the cell's ability to take in and store energy, like proteins, fats, and glucose.

called "blood sugar") levels. A more accurate view of the same issue would scrutinize insulin. During insulin resistance, the compromised insulin action on tissues like muscle results in the muscle having a harder time pulling in glucose from the blood. As a result, blood glucose levels start to rise over time.

If we looked at blood insulin levels, we could actually detect the problem years, even decades, before the glucose levels ever rise.[2] Because blood insulin levels would have already been climbing for years due to underlying unrecognized insulin resistance.

The constellation of markers listed above—waist circumference, blood glucose, blood pressure, and disordered blood lipids—constitute the metabolic syndrome, which you've almost certainly heard of. However, "metabolic syndrome" is simply the latest term for a long-known trend of these seemingly distinct issues occurring together. One of its earlier names, and one that is far more descriptive and revealing of the true problem, was the "insulin resistance syndrome."[3]

This matters a great deal. As striking as it is to realize the role insulin resistance plays in causing or contributing to several chronic diseases (as mentioned in the introduction), the prevalence of insulin resistance provides additional, and sobering, context. Insulin resistance has become the most common health disorder in the world, and it affects almost all adults in the United States.[4] But it is too often misdiagnosed or outright overlooked.

So, before you put the book down, thinking you're among the healthy (insulin-sensitive) 12%, don't be so quick. As I've stated: insulin resistance is very often undiagnosed, and even the five complications listed above are far from an exhaustive list. And even if you *are* insulin sensitive, well, you might still benefit from the information throughout and especially at the end of this book.

To help us start to find out where you are, let's take a quick quiz (after all, nothing delights a professor like Ben more than a pop quiz!):

* Have you been told you have hypertension?
* Do you have family members who have had type 2 diabetes or gestational diabetes?

- Do you have any particular skin disorders, such as dark, rough skin around your neck, or little skin tags around your neck?
- For women, do you have PCOS? For men, do you have erectile dysfunction or "low testosterone"?

This list seems random, but each of these problems is related to, either cause or consequence of, insulin resistance, as elaborated in *Why We Get Sick*. Of course, these are far from conclusive, but they're surprisingly telling. (The results of this quiz are on page 17, if you just need to skip ahead and find out!)

A version of this quiz appears in *Why We Get Sick,* and it's a solid starting point. But let's explore some other ways you can get a clearer idea of where you stand regarding insulin resistance—lab tests and even some DIY methods to determine where you are metabolically.

Ranges in the following test results have been given a score of 1 to 3. Several of these tests are readily available as part of a standard blood panel, especially the lipid-based tests (triglycerides, HDL cholesterol, etc.); of course, the results of these tests you'll receive from the lab or your doctor will be reported in a range of different units. So the score of 1 to 3 is simply a method to create a consistent scoring across the various blood tests (a way of comparing apples to oranges and still getting relevant results, if you will).

Elevated insulin, stress, and inflammation are the primary drivers of insulin resistance. We'll explore those causes in later chapters.

If you're able to get the tests performed, you'll have a great idea of how to apply the principles and paths laid out later in the book. To be clear, we're assuming that you won't get *all* of these tests (although you certainly could if you wanted to). Even if you can get only one or two of the tests, the scoring from 1 to 3 will still be helpful. And if you can't get any of the tests, you can use a DIY method or even the pop quiz results to determine your path forward.

Insulin-Based Tests

The first category of tests measures that often-overlooked (but obvious) metric—insulin—by itself and in combination with other factors.

Fasting insulin

The first test is simply measuring insulin itself—a pretty obvious choice if you want to understand something called insulin resistance. Despite this, insulin has been so broadly overlooked that there's never been a general consensus on what insulin levels should be. Thankfully, there are enough studies that we can make sound conclusions.

If your fasting insulin (i.e., insulin after you haven't eaten for about 6 hours) is less than ~6 microunits per milliliter of blood (μU/mL), you're in good shape and likely insulin sensitive. This gets you a **score of 1**.

You fall into the intermediate range of likely being insulin resistant if you have a fasting insulin of 7 to 17 μU/mL. This range is a bit broader to account for the fact that insulin, like most hormones, has an ebb and flow—it can rise and fall slightly throughout the day. This range helps account for that, but it still matters. A person with 8 μU/mL has double the risk of developing type 2 diabetes as a person with 5 μU/mL.[5] In this range, you get a **score of 2**.

If your insulin is in the high teens and beyond (18+ μU/mL), you should be worried. At that level, you are likely insulin resistant and might have even noticed symptoms of it, such as hypertension or infertility. If you're here, you **score a 3**.

Interpreting Your Fasting Insulin Results

Your Results	Your Score
<6 μU/mL	1
7-17 μU/mL	2
18+ μU/mL	3

To get a fasting insulin test, you will often need to explicitly request it from your clinician, or get it done through an independent clinical lab service.

Homeostatic model assessment (HOMA)

In this assessment, we look at both fasting insulin and fasting glucose. This is a match made in heaven—insulin and glucose are so intimately connected in

> Insulin has been so broadly overlooked that there's never been a general consensus on what insulin levels should be.

the body that it only makes sense to keep them connected when we measure them both clinically.

To figure it out, just take:

$$[\textbf{Glucose (mg/dL)} \times \textbf{Insulin (μU/L)}] \,/\, \textbf{405}$$

A value under 1.5 is an indicator of insulin sensitivity (**1 point**), and above 4 usually means you're borderline type 2 diabetic (**3 points**). If your number is 1.6 to 3.9, you're in the middle (and get **2 points**).

Interpreting Your HOMA Results

Your Results	Your Score
<1.5	1
1.6–3.9	2
4+	3

Adipose-IR (adipo-IR)

This is a newer test, recently described in a handful of studies. Before we get to the test, let's pause to cover the justification for it (because it's just so neat).

Fat cells are designed to store fat for later use, and fat gets broken down when the body needs energy, in a process called "lipolysis." When a fat cell breaks down fat, it releases the fat as a "free fatty acid" (FFA), which can then be used for energy by tissues throughout the body, such as muscles, bones, and more. This happens anytime insulin is low, because insulin abhors breaking down fat. Insulin wages war on fat metabolism by attacking the process at multiple fronts, including at the very origin—the fat cell (we'll come back to this later). That means the two variables—insulin and FFA—should never be elevated at the same time. Either insulin is high (which inhibits fat breakdown from the fat cell) and FFA are low, or insulin is low (which allows fat breakdown at fat cells) and FFA are high. Unless, that is, the fat cells are insulin resistant.

There is compelling evidence that fat cells are the first relevant cells to become insulin resistant (a case laid out in *Why We Get Sick*). This means the adipo-IR score could be your first glimpse into whether you're becoming insulin resistant. The formula is:

$$\textbf{insulin (μU/mL)} \times \textbf{FFA (mmol/L)}$$

Because males and females have different rates of fat burning in response to insulin (women naturally burn more fat), there are different categories. You have insulin-sensitive fat cells if your adipo-IR score is <5 for men or <8 for women (**1 point**). A score of 5 to 10 (men) or 8 to 16 (women) suggests something is going wrong (**2 points**), and anything higher is a strong indicator that your fat cells have succumbed to insulin resistance (**3 points**).

Interpreting Your Adipo-IR Results

Your Results		Your Score
Male	Female	
<5	<8	1
5-10	8-16	2
10+	16+	3

Dynamic insulin

This last insulin-related test is the best, but it's the most difficult to get done because you need to be in a place where you can get your blood drawn at least four times. Generally, this happens at a clinic. The word *dynamic* means that insulin is measured repeatedly in a short window of time (about 2 hours) to get an idea of how it responds to a challenge. In short, the way this test is performed is to drink a small cup of pure glucose and get your blood drawn immediately, and again roughly every 30 minutes for 2 hours, to measure insulin.[6]

The best outcome is for your highest point ("peak") to be at 30 minutes and not get higher than about 60μU/mL (**1 point**). The next best result is to have a peak that stays below 60 μU/mL but occurs at a time point later than 30 minutes (i.e., 60, 90, 120 minutes; **2 points**). The worst outcome is when everything is elevated—your insulin is higher than 60 μU/mL at 30 minutes and remains elevated (>30μU/mL) at 2 hours (**3 points**).

Interpreting Your Dynamic Insulin Results

Your Results		Your Score
Peak value	Peak time	
Below 60 μU/mL at 30 minutes and below 30 μU/mL at 2 hours	30 minutes	1
Below 60 μU/mL at 30 minutes and below 30 μU/mL at 2 hours	60, 90, or 120 minutes	2
Above 60 μU/mL at 30 minutes or above 30 μU/mL at 2 hours	Any time, but above the cutoff	3

Blood Lipid Tests

The next tests scrutinize blood lipids, especially fasting triglycerides.

Triglycerides are a storage form of fat, though in this case, that fat is not "stored" but rather traveling through the blood (this is a blood test, after all). Triglycerides are carried through the blood, either from the diet or freshly produced by the liver, on lipoproteins, particularly chylomicrons (from the food we just ate) or very-low-density/low-density lipoproteins (VLDL/LDL) made by the liver. Of course, in a fasted state, there won't be any triglycerides from the diet, so we get only a measurement of what the liver is making, which is relevant because insulin has a powerful influence over this process.

Insulin stimulates the liver to make fat from glucose and further instructs the liver to package these individual fats into packs of three—that's the "tri-" in "triglycerides"—before shipping out on a lipoprotein. Thus, if insulin is high, as it is with insulin resistance, triglycerides will be elevated, which makes it a sensitive marker of insulin resistance. This marker can be used in two helpful scores.

Triglyceride-glucose index

The triglyceride-glucose (TyG) index combines triglycerides (TG) with an obvious culprit in glucose. Because insulin increases TG but decreases glucose, the two variables shouldn't be elevated at the same time. That's what the TyG reveals.

The formula is complicated, unfortunately, but a calculator can make quick work of it:

$$\ln* \left[\textbf{fasting TGs (mg/dL)} \times \textbf{fasting glucose (mg/dL)}/\textbf{2} \right]$$

It's that "ln" or "natural logarithm" that makes things a bit tricky, at least for most of us—after all, it's probably been a while since high school algebra. After you multiply the TG and glucose, divide by 2, then hit the "ln" button. That will give you the required index number.[7] If the TyG is under 4.5, that's a great score (**1 point**). If you get 4.6 to 5, that's OK (**2 points**), but any higher than 5 is a problem (**3 points**).

Interpreting Your TyG

Your Results	Your Score
<4.5	1
4.6–5	2
5+	3

Triglyceride-HDL cholesterol ratio

The TG:HDL ratio (dividing TG by HDL) is a commonly used measurement of insulin resistance for reasons that are similar to the TyG—like TG, HDL cholesterol is impacted by insulin.

While insulin has a general activating effect with cholesterol production in the liver, its effect on the lipoproteins that carry the cholesterol are varied. Insulin activates the production of VLDL, which helps the liver move its newly produced cholesterol out of the liver and into circulation. However, HDL, which is generally bringing cholesterol *back* to the liver, works against insulin's desire to move cholesterol *out*. It's no surprise, then, that chronically elevated insulin lowers HDL cholesterol.

The net effect of insulin resistance is to generally increase TG and reduce HDL, resulting in an ever-increasing TG:HDL ratio. One wrinkle with the TG:HDL ratio is that it changes across ethnicities, resulting in different cut-offs that make it difficult to create a single cutoff that can apply to everyone. In White and Asian people, a TG:HDL ratio of 1.5 is reliably good, but this number is a little higher in Hispanic people (closer to 2) and a little lower in African American people (closer to 1).[8]

Accordingly, we need to give the TG:HDL ratio less weight than the other tests and simplify the scoring. If your TG:HDL ratio is less than 2, it's a generally good sign (**1 point**), but above this, it could reflect a problem (**2 points**).

Interpreting Your TG:HDL Ratio

Your Results	Your Score
<2	1
2+	2

Where Are You?

Up to this point, we've looked at two methods you can lean on to see where you are on the spectrum of insulin resistance: the quiz and the clinical tests. Let's collect your scores.

1. ***Insulin sensitive:*** You are the fortunate few who answered "no" to all the quiz questions, and/or had 1s across the board in the clinical tests—you're among that healthy 12% of the average adult population. You're doing great. Insulin is working very well throughout your body and your insulin levels are in a healthy low range. Your primary motivation with this book is either to stay where you are and prevent insulin resistance, or to learn how you can help friends or family. In general, your path is going to be more liberal than the others, but it's guided enough to help you stay on track; you'll follow the Maintain path.

2. ***Mildly insulin resistant:*** This is a complicated group because it includes two distinct populations. On the one hand, this group includes those who are currently only mildly insulin resistant (a couple of 2s in the lab tests, but mostly 1s)—perhaps you're catching this right on the edge of the rapidly descending and slippery slope to insulin resistance. On the other hand, this group also includes those who have clawed themselves back up that slippery slope (i.e., have all 1s and a couple of 2s now, but used to have plenty of 2s and 3s). You know what it's like to win the metabolic fight. This plan is then both offense (for those wanting to improve) and defense (for those wanting to keep their hard-earned gains). Or, you answered "yes" to one of the quiz questions. (However, there's some nuance about *which* quiz question. If your "yes" was to having high blood pressure, it's a tenuous membership—there are other, though less common, causes of hypertension. In contrast, if your "yes" was in response to having PCOS, gestational diabetes, or skin tags, it's a much more certain inclusion into this group. Not all "yesses" are created equal.) Preventing your insulin resistance from becoming more critical will require some commitment to dietary and exercise changes; you'll follow the Prevent path.

3. ***Fully insulin resistant:*** You answered "yes" to two or more of the quiz questions (the more "yesses," the more work lies ahead) and/or got a 3 in

your clinical test results. You are further along the spectrum of insulin resistance and will need to be more determined to reverse course and work your way to the opposite end of the spectrum. Don't worry—we have the plan to get you there. You'll follow the Reverse path.

Throughout this book, we can't help but use the analogy of a slippery slope. If you're looking to reverse insulin resistance, you will implement the strategies outlined in the chapters that follow to ascend the slope back toward insulin sensitivity. If you're hoping to prevent insulin resistance, you're aiming

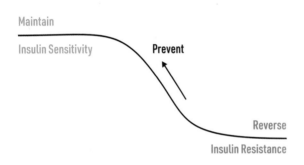

not to slide down to insulin resistance, especially if you just got out of it; we have a plan to help. And lastly, in the event you're already insulin sensitive, you want to continue to enjoy the view from the metabolic summit. You don't have as much work, but it still requires a diligent and deliberate plan to stay there.

The Wrinkle of Age

Quiz and clinical test scores might be straightforward, but we need to acknowledge an additional factor: aging. Nobody will be surprised to learn that there are numerous metabolic consequences of getting old.

Science has long known that the older we get, the more insulin resistance settles in. This simply and unfortunately means that the results of the clinical tests described in this chapter are likelier to be 2s and 3s the older you get. However, by understanding the reasons why this happens, you can fight the trend much, much better and keep your "mature" body insulin sensitive longer than otherwise.

One of the most important variables with aging and insulin resistance is what happens to our tissues. Skeletal muscle and fat tissue are the two largest insulin-responsive tissues in the average person. As we age, we tend to lose muscle and gain fat in a particularly unfortunate way. Nevertheless, if your muscle and fat are insulin sensitive, then you are insulin sensitive.

With muscle and fat, it's all about size . . . but in totally opposite ways.

Muscle is a powerful metabolic tool for a few reasons. In addition to its high mass in the body, it has a high metabolic rate with a high glucose consumption—it's the "lion's share" glucose eater in the body. When insulin climbs, almost all of the glucose that leaves the blood goes into muscle.

The older we get, the more our muscles shrink. To a degree, some of this is due to irreversible changes in hormones, like growth hormone and testosterone, which make it harder for the body to keep its muscle mass. However, the other (enormous) cause of this muscle loss is mechanics and disuse—we simply stop moving our muscles like we used to.

Tragically, this problem becomes self-perpetuating. As the muscles become insulin resistant, they also lose the benefit of insulin itself. Insulin doesn't stimulate muscle growth as much as it defends it—insulin wants the muscle to keep all its protein inside. But again, when the muscle can't respond to insulin as well, we start to lose muscle mass.

> Insulin doesn't stimulate muscle growth as much as it defends it—insulin wants the muscle to keep all its protein inside.

In the end, as we lose muscle mass (mostly by shrinking muscle cells), we lose the largest glucose consumer, which means we have a harder time lowering glucose when insulin is trying to push it out of the blood. Ultimately, this forces insulin to stay higher for longer as it tries to find other suitable places for the glucose. Enter the fat cell . . .

The effect of aging on fat cells is fascinating. We humans have a remarkable ability to store fat (unlike most mammals) and we do it very well through infancy and childhood. Indeed, during these stages and through adolescence, we actively *make new fat cells*—our actual fat cell number is increasing during this time. However, with the end of adolescence comes the end of fat-cell producing potential (usually). That means that the number of fat cells we have as we enter adulthood is generally the number of fat cells we keep.[9] If we gain or lose fat during adulthood, it's largely a matter of growing or shrinking of the fat cells, not so much a matter gaining or losing fat cells. But things change when we get older.

As we enter the latter quarter of life (60+ years), things start working in reverse; whereas our childhood was spent making new fat cells, our older years are spent losing them. On the surface, this sounds like a good thing. You're probably thinking, *Who wouldn't want to lose fat cells?* It's what happens *because* of the lost fat cells that's a problem.

Testing at Home

There are other tools you might be able to use at home to see which metabolic neighborhood you're in at the moment. They don't require a formal visit to the clinic but are more direct than the quiz.

Continuous glucose monitor:

Insulin's best-known effect (but far from its only job!) is to control blood glucose. When glucose rises in the blood, it can be lethal in short order if it stays high; insulin is the primary mechanism to lower glucose by essentially opening access into numerous body cells, like muscle and fat cells, and escorting the glucose out of the blood and into those cells. But don't fall into the glucose-based trap! Remember (from *Why We Get Sick*) that relying on glucose leads to ill-formed conclusions—glucose levels can be normal in insulin resistance, and clinical interventions aimed at lowering glucose by pushing up insulin make everything worse.

Modern tools allow us to measure glucose at every moment of the day. It's in this *dynamic* capacity of a continuous glucose monitor (CGM) where glucose really becomes helpful in measuring insulin resistance.

There are two useful things to pay attention to if you are able to wear a CGM. First, the more you see glucose levels oscillating (large swings up and down) throughout the day, the more likely it is you have insulin resistance.[1] If your glucose levels have modest swings, it's a good sign of insulin sensitivity.

For the second, you can conduct a test on yourself. Starting from a fast wherein glucose levels are stable, eat two large pieces of bread. If your glucose levels rise and then get back to below 100 mg/dL in 2 hours, it's pretty good evidence that you are insulin sensitive. One important note with this: if you adhere to a low-carbohydrate diet normally, you may get a false positive—you might "fail" the test even if you're very insulin sensitive. When the pancreas gets the sense that it doesn't need to produce as much insulin as it used to, it keeps less insulin "on hand." When all of a sudden you eat a lot of carbohydrates, it simply takes the pancreas a little longer than normal to make the required insulin, which manifests as a longer-than-normal glucose curve. The solution is simple: just warn the pancreas ahead of time that a load is coming by eating more carbohydrates the day before.

1   Hall, H., et al. *Glucotypes reveal new patterns of glucose dysregulation.* PLoS Biol, 2018. **16**(7): p. e2005143.

Ketone meter:

There are few topics more polarizing than ketones. These much-maligned and misunderstood molecules are actually metabolic heavyweights, reducing inflammation and fueling cells, including cells in the brain. Beyond their effects, it's what they reflect that we want to focus on—when ketones are detectable, insulin is low.

Insulin controls fuel metabolism in the body by dictating what cells are able to do with nutrients. When insulin is elevated, it promotes cellular processes that result in nutrients rushing into cells and being used either to create other molecules or to be stored for later use. When insulin is low, it does the opposite—cells are now disassembling molecules, usually to increase nutrients in the blood. Basically, if insulin is high, cells are storing energy; when insulin is low, cells are burning energy.

One of the most powerful nutrient-specific effects of insulin is its control of fat metabolism, which is where ketones come in. When insulin is low, fat cells start breaking down stored fat to release into the blood, and the body starts burning fat as a fuel at a much higher rate. As this fat burning continues for several hours (again, as insulin is kept low), it's almost as if the body is burning more fat than it needs—the cells have enough energy—but fat burning can't stop because insulin is still low. This "extra" fat burning becomes ketones. That's right—ketones are simply products of high fat burning. Because this process is totally controlled by insulin, ketones can be viewed as an *inverse indicator* of insulin levels. If ketones are high, that means insulin is low.

To leverage this biochemical reality into something useful, you can measure ketones to get an idea of where your insulin levels are. There are numerous ways to measure ketones, including from the breath, urine, and blood. The latter is of course the most accurate, but it's the least comfortable (finger prick tests are no fun). Ketone meters can be purchased at many drug stores and through numerous online retailers.

To get an idea of where your insulin levels are at, try fasting for 24 hours (no calories in). At the end of the fast, if your ketone meter indicates ketones at around 0.3 mM or higher, it's very strong evidence that your insulin levels are at a healthy low level, and low insulin suggests an insulin-sensitive state. In contrast, if you have insulin resistance, even after fasting your insulin levels will likely be high enough to inhibit ketogenesis. This would lead to ketones being lower than the level indicated and likely below the level of detection. So no ketones after fasting indicates insulin resistance.

Diana's Motivation

My biggest motivation to learn about nutrition was to teach my children. It's no secret that the younger generations are beginning to experience chronic diseases, like obesity and diabetes, at alarming rates. We owe it to our kids to correct our own eating and lifestyle habits to model how to eat the way the human body was designed to eat.

The stakes are high . . . it's life and death. It's also about quality of life, getting to enjoy experiences, and living with a sense of bodily well-being. All of that is so close within your reach—all you have to do is reach out and claim it for yourself.

If an older person were to start to lose fat cells because of age, but continued to eat the same way that put that amount of fat on the body in the first place, the body won't lose *fat*—it simply shifts it, so the remaining fat cells are forced to carry the metabolic load. That means they grow, which is not ideal. This is a process called hypertrophy, where each individual fat cell gets larger—as if the fat cells become overfat. Having overfat fat cells may sound silly, but it's really at the heart of insulin resistance.

Fat cells are capable of remarkable growth—they can grow well over 10 times their original (normal) size. This individual fat cell growth is what accounts for the overwhelming majority of fat gain a person experiences. Unfortunately, as the fat cell reaches its maximum potential size, it becomes metabolically problematic in the body in two ways, but it does so all in an effort to save itself.

Firstly, it needs to stop growing. The fat cell knows (in a way) that if it continues to respond to insulin, the overwhelmingly primary signal to grow, it will burst. Insulin mostly signals a fat cell to grow by limiting the fat cell's ability to break down fat. Thus, in order to prevent further growth, the fat cell becomes less sensitive (i.e., resistant) to insulin's efforts. So even though insulin is trying to promote further growth by inhibiting lipolysis (i.e., the breakdown of fat in the fat cell), the fat cell isn't responding, and it can begin breaking down its stored fats. This results in higher than expected blood FFA (per the adipo-IR score mentioned earlier).

At the same time that the fat cells are growing ever larger, they need ever more access to blood. As the fat cells enlarge, they begin pushing each other farther and farther away from capillaries and the life-giving nutrients and oxygen they provide. In order to not "suffocate" (or, more accurately, become "hypoxic"—a low oxygen state), the expanded fat cells produce and release cytokines, small pro-inflammatory proteins that can stimulate the growth of new blood vessels. However, these cytokines have a nasty side: some of them just move around the body and activate inflammation.

Collectively, these two events—increased FFA and elevated inflammation—promote insulin resistance throughout the body. But it all started with the expanded fat cells trying to ensure their own survival. And in this context, it all started with someone simply getting older. (Hypertrophy can also result from eating certain types of fats, which we will explore in chapter 4.)

One final and critical metabolic problem with getting old is sleep. The older we get, the worse we sleep. This is more than just having a lot on your mind—there are genuine changes in the brain and the production of sleep hormones, like melatonin, that lead to unavoidable sleep changes.[10] As we will see in chapter 7, sleep has a powerful metabolic influence—one bad night of sleep results in demonstrable insulin resistance the next day.[11] Considering the years of "bad nights" that come with sleeping more poorly with age, it's little surprise that age-related sleep changes contribute to a greater struggle with maintaining insulin resistance.

> Know this: it is entirely possible to reverse and prevent insulin resistance with aging, and the strategies outlined in later chapters will work very well.

Before the discouragement grows too much, know this: it is entirely possible to reverse and prevent insulin resistance with aging, and the strategies outlined in later chapters will work very well. The dietary and meal planning strategies apply regardless of age. The exercise component, however, shifts appropriately with age.

The older we get, the more we worry about injury, and injury usually comes with heavy weights or fast movements. Thus, the exercises outlined later in the book can be tailored to account for older joints that prefer more gentle movements, especially with resistance exercise (such as weight training). More important than the amount of weight is that the movement is performed enough to "fail." In other words, you can perform an exercise with a relatively lighter weight, but repeat the exercise to the point that you can't comfortably do any more[12] (more on this later).

An important takeaway regarding aging and insulin resistance is that the older we get, the more careful we need to be. Of course, it's very possible to be 75 years old and perfectly insulin sensitive, but it's less likely than when that same person was 25 years old. Given the trend, even if you're insulin sensitive based

Ben on Myths and Misunderstandings of Physiological Insulin Resistance

When I started writing *Why We Get Sick* a number of years ago, I was one of very few voices speaking about the dangers of insulin resistance, including what it is, where it comes from, and what to do about it. As the space has become more crowded, with many new voices joining the chorus, some prominent soloists are inadvertently singing a different tune. The aberrant anthem is simple: a low-carbohydrate diet causes physiological insulin resistance.

Not all insulin resistance is bad. My focus as a scientist and author has been on pathological (i.e., harmful) insulin resistance—the insulin resistance that is a result of harmful stimuli (poor diet, poor sleep, etc.) and causes harmful problems (diabetes, dementia, etc.). Another area of expertise for me, however, is a lesser-known context of insulin resistance when it serves a good purpose—physiological (i.e., helpful) insulin resistance. Unfortunately, physiological insulin resistance is often discussed in wholly incorrect ways.

Physiological insulin resistance is caused by growth-stimulating hormones that climb considerably during the "2 Ps" of human life: puberty and pregnancy. What these two states have in common is growth—the body needs to grow in certain ways. In puberty, the growth is obvious—the child grows bigger and taller. For this to happen, growth hormone itself, which comes from the brain, is the insulin antagonist that drives the insulin resistance. In pregnancy, the mother is growing fat and mammary tissue, as well as helping the baby grow larger; a related growth hormone, a version that comes from the placenta, drives the insulin resistance.

There is no dietary cause of physiological insulin resistance. Those who say a low-carb diet can create it mistake *glucose intolerance* for *insulin resistance*.

Glucose intolerance is a state in which the body has a hard time clearing glucose from the blood and moving it into cells. As an example, let's look at the oral glucose tolerance test we discussed earlier. In the following figure, you can see that in glucose intolerance, it takes longer for the glucose curve to settle down, relative to the glucose-tolerant state.

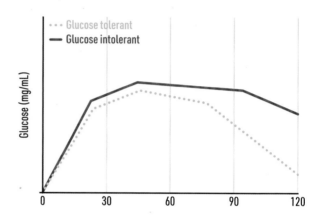

Very often, this is a function of insulin resistance. Obviously, if a body is insulin resistant, insulin is less capable of lowering glucose (mostly less capable of pushing the glucose into muscle, but other tissues, as well), and it thus takes longer for the glucose to drop. At the same time, insulin is higher for longer—as the insulin isn't working as well, the body needs more. But there's another explanation for glucose intolerance that is almost the opposite of insulin resistance. As shown in the following figure, if we superimpose insulin, the picture becomes clearer (though a little complicated at first glance).

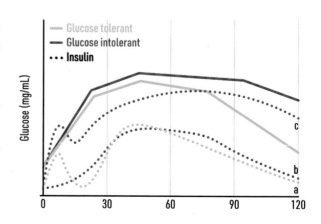

When insulin is released in response to a rise in glucose, it comes in two phases. The first phase is a function of the pancreatic beta cells releasing insulin that it already has on hand—that is, insulin it made earlier and kept ready for when it was needed urgently (such as after eating a bunch of glucose). The second phase consists of the pancreas making *new* insulin on demand; naturally, this part takes longer, but it also allows the pancreas to fine-tune the glucose with real-time feedback to ensure glucose returns to normal in good order. But the beta cells are efficient—they don't like to keep insulin around if it isn't needed. That's why in as little as a 24-hour fast, the beta cells disassemble the premade insulin, thinking it's simply not needed anymore. The same applies to a low-carbohydrate diet—if the body isn't eating glucose often, why keep all that insulin around?

Any form of insulin resistance, whether pathological or physiological, will result in glucose intolerance (the solid orange line) with elevated insulin (dotted orange line "c") relative to a normal glucose-tolerant, insulin-sensitive state (solid blue line; dotted blue line "a"). You'll notice that in these two states, insulin secretion has both phases—the rapid first phase (within minutes) and the much larger second phase (over the next hour or so).

As noted above, a low-carbohydrate diet and even a modest fast result in the *temporary* loss of the first phase of insulin secretion (dotted orange line "b"), but a normal second phase.[1] This is a unique state—the body is *insulin sensitive, but glucose intolerant*. If you want the first phase of insulin back (perhaps because you want to eat carbohydrates more often or you need to pass a clinical glucose tolerance test), then you simply eat some amount of carbohydrate a few hours before. With this, the beta cells get the message that insulin is needed more frequently, and they build up a store of insulin to accommodate the demands in the future (i.e., first phase is back).

1   Jorgensen, S. W., et al. *Impact of prolonged fasting on insulin secretion, insulin action, and hepatic versus whole body insulin secretion disposition indices in healthy young males.* Am J Physiol Endocrinol Metab, 2021. **320**(2): p. E281-90.

on the markers discussed earlier, and would thus normally be in the "maintain" category, it would be prudent to consider the strategies in the "prevent" category.

Now that you know which path you'll follow throughout this book, it's time to focus on the principles—the science behind the eating and exercise guidelines to follow. Since we've mentioned fasting throughout this chapter, let's start there: When should you eat?

Watch the Clock

Fasting is a remarkably effective and powerful strategy to lower insulin and improve insulin sensitivity. Insulin is simply antithetical to fasting; insulin is the hormone of the "fed state." This concept was established and heavily emphasized by the work of Dr. George Cahill, a legendary scientist who studied the human responses to fasting (we mention him by name in the hopes that some of you will look deeper into his fascinating work).

If insulin is the hormone of the fed state, then what we eat matters. The three macronutrients—carbohydrates, proteins, and fats—have disparate effects on insulin, with carbohydrates having the greatest effect. (Of course, the specific effect can vary greatly within those categories—for instance, let's consider two foods that are primarily carbohydrate; insulin release is practically nonexistent with broccoli, but it's substantial with candy.) But most meals will be a mix of macronutrients, which nevertheless results in some degree of insulin secretion.

On its own, this isn't overly problematic (though the mix of macros does matter, and we'll look at that in the next chapter). But it's the timing that becomes a challenge.

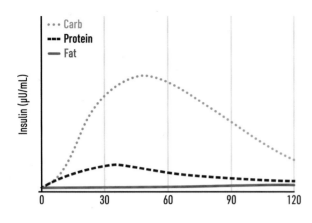

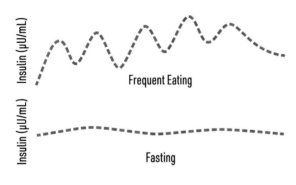

The average individual eats the wrong foods and eats them *too often*. Depending on the food consumed, and the inherent insulin sensitivity of the person, it can take insulin over three hours to return to normal levels. Because our culture is one of constant eating and snacking, the average person spends *all waking moments in a state of elevated insulin*. By the time insulin starts to come down overnight, we immediately break that brief nighttime fast by starting the day with insulin-spiking foods (indeed, the typical American breakfast may be the worst meal of the day in this regard).

This chronically elevated insulin is a primary driver of insulin resistance. Yes, too much insulin causes insulin resistance. This biological fact has been shown to exist in all three biomedical research models—isolated cells, animals, and humans. Want to make cells stop responding to insulin? Add extra insulin into the cell culture bath. Want to make laboratory rodents insulin resistant? Just infuse some extra insulin. You get the idea. The same applies to humans.

The solution with fasting is wonderfully simple: when we don't eat or drink anything but water, insulin stays low and the body becomes more sensitive to it.

In fact, even people with such profound insulin resistance that they have type 2 diabetes and require drugs to keep their glucose in a decent range are able to reverse their insulin resistance with intermittent fasting, and to such a degree that they no longer need any medications![1]

Though fasting itself is simple, it's become a little complicated in recent years as people seek to find a way to implement a strategy that works. When looking at the data on eating frequency, two timing factors stand out—how the person eats *daily* and how the person eats *monthly*. In the longer time frame, people who fast roughly 6 to 10 times per year (for 24 hours) have about 50% as much chance of developing insulin resistance as people who don't fast.[2]

Moreover, eating less frequently in a given day, rather than multiple smaller meals, leads to greater insulin sensitivity.[3]

Time-Restricted Eating

For convenience, many people prefer to leverage a time-restricted eating pattern, in which they structure their eating to occur within a specific period of time in a day. This might look like fasting for 23 hours and then eating one meal a day (or what people call "OMAD") or, more often, two meals a day, with a fast overnight and when a third meal would usually occur. The timing of the eating window can change.

> The solution with fasting is wonderfully simple: when we don't eat or drink anything but water, insulin stays low and the body becomes more sensitive to it.

When compared head to head, eating early is better than eating late.[4] In other words, eating breakfast and lunch, but fasting through dinner, is better than fasting through breakfast, then eating lunch and dinner. Of course, this is terrible timing; not eating dinner is a great way to make every evening with friends and family awkward (and bringing a pitcher of water to a potluck won't win you any friends).

Many people find it easier to fast through breakfast—they're just not hungry in the morning. We would never advise anyone to eat when they're not hungry! What's more, there's good reason to consider restricting particularly carbohydrates in the morning due to something called the dawn phenomenon.

Our hormones naturally ebb and flow throughout the day. Some of these hormones (including insulin itself) have an effect on insulin sensitivity. Every morning, insulin levels start to climb around 5:30 a.m. and drop back down within about two hours.[5] This is known as the "dawn phenomenon" or "dawn effect." To test how powerful it is, a science team had research subjects drink glucose three times throughout the day. In response to the drink, insulin spiked the highest in the morning and lowest in the evening;[6] in fact, in the morning it was almost twice as high!

One reason for this is the work of hormones that counter insulin's actions, most especially cortisol. These anti-insulin hormones climb in the morning, as they seek to increase blood glucose.[7] Naturally, the higher these hormones are, the more resistant to insulin the body becomes.

Because of this, eating a starchy/sugary meal in the morning potentially carries a greater metabolic burden than eating that same meal any other time of day.[8] Taken all together, more important than timing is the composition of *what* you eat, rather than *when* you eat.

As mentioned in the previous chapter, insulin resistance likely begins in enlarged fat cells. But while the *body* becomes a little insulin resistant in the morning, fat cells go the other way; fat tissue is *more insulin sensitive* in the morning and less so in the evening.[9] This is a wicked metabolic combination. Because insulin inhibits fat burning[10] and, in contrast, promotes fat cell growth,[11] eating an insulin-spiking food in the morning could carry an enhanced fat-promoting effect that leads to a vicious cycle.

Between these two perspectives, there may be a good compromise. Skipping breakfast, eating a big lunch, and then having a modest dinner relatively early in the evening and nothing thereafter is a great way to implement some degree of fasting into your lifestyle plan. With this strategy, insulin sensitivity can improve rapidly.[12]

One wrinkle with this plan is the "eating nothing after dinner" in the evening. Without a doubt, that is when people appear to be at their weakest—the witching hour of snacking. There could be something in your fridge or cupboard that hasn't tempted you even slightly all day, but once evening comes around, the temptation grows and grows. You must have a plan to deal with this. For Ben, the simplest strategy has been to simply not have those kinds of snacks in the home. Willpower can be stronger at the grocery store than it is at home in the evenings. You can also try drinking a little pickle juice or some apple cider vinegar, or simply drinking more water (maybe with a little salt). A salty/bitter kick to the taste buds can take the edge off an evening craving. If you're too hungry and just gotta have *something*, a snack that won't spike insulin is the next best choice (we'll cover what those are in the next chapters, and you'll find some recipes in chapter 13).

Day Fasting

For those who want to fast on the order of 24 hours and more, do so smartly and planned, with an emphasis on hydration and minerals. As with time-restricted eating, this can take multiple forms, but three are primary:

1. **Alternate day fasting:** you eat normally one day, then fast the next.
2. **5-2 fasting:** you eat normally for five days, then fast for two days straight.
3. **Once-weekly fasting:** you eat normally for six days in a week and fast for one day. (This works especially well on Mondays, after a potentially indulgent weekend, and it's easy to stick with.)

One challenge with daylong fasts is avoiding a vicious cycle of mounting hunger followed by overindulgence. This form of "fasting" is really an eating disorder—a glamorized version of a binge-purge pattern. The best way to avoid this is to ensure you have a solid plan for *ending* your fast. If it's helpful, look at the fast as actually going *longer* than you think. For example, rather than just ending a fast at 24 hours, think of that 24-hour fast as actually being a 30-hour fast—you avoid calories for 24 hours, but then you deliberately have a specific food or drink at that 24-hour mark that helps maintain the low insulin from the fasting (e.g., a food or drink enriched with protein and fat), then follow that up a few hours later with something else. *How you end a fast matters much more than how long you fast!*

There are several cautionary notes with regard to day fasts. An obvious one is that fasting should be avoided if a person has a history of an eating disorder

Fasting and Sleep

One of the most important habits that can help improve metabolic health is getting good sleep (we'll revisit this topic in chapter 7). Sleep can be an elusive bedfellow for reasons that are often beyond our control, but thankfully, there is one important step you can take: keeping glucose under control before going to bed.

One of the leading causes of insomnia is elevated body temperature.[1] We have long known that people with diabetes tend to have a higher body temperature when glucose is elevated,[2] an effect that is exacerbated by exercise.[3] What we know now is that it's the glucose—when glucose is high, body temperature is too, even in people without diabetes.[4]

Because of this, eating or drinking a glucose-spiking meal or snack before bed will often result in elevated body temperature and subsequent insomnia.[5] Try to prevent this and get a good night of sleep by ensuring no snacking in the evening, or at least no snacking that spikes your glucose. Easier said than done—glucose-spiking treats are what we're drawn to. Few people sit around in the evening and crave a plate of bacon and eggs; we want something sweet and gooey or salty and crunchy, which means something rich in refined carbohydrates. Aside from the salty/bitter drinks mentioned earlier, the recipe chapter in this book has some excellent options for snacks that won't spike glucose.

like anorexia nervosa or bulimia. Second, the leaner the body, the more cautious you need to be with fasting. There's a fine line between fasting and starvation, and that line is . . . fat.

> **Our bodies are designed to be able to take prolonged breaks from food.**

When you start to run low on fat tissue (a problem admittedly few people face), your brain is put in a difficult situation. When you start to fast, your brain becomes a hybrid engine. In the average individual, eating mostly carbohydrates, the brain relies almost wholly on glucose as its fuel source. But with fasting or a low-carbohydrate diet, glucose becomes sparse and insulin becomes low. With the lower insulin comes an increase in fat metabolism, and when fat metabolism is increased, ketones are made. This is the brain's cue to shift its fuel use from glucose to ketones, which the brain does gladly—even when ketones are at a lower level in the blood than glucose, the brain has already started using ketones at a higher rate. This happy metabolic state can continue as long as there is fat on the body to make ketones. When fat starts to run low, ketones do too, at which point the brain is forced to shift back to glucose, but this time it comes at a cost—the liver makes the glucose from amino acids stripped from the muscle protein. Your fat tissue is *the* critical defender that differentiates a fast from starvation, and after that, muscle acts as the final fuel source to keep the brain going.

As with day fasts, it's important to be smart about what you eat when you finish a multiple-day fast. Years ago, scientists who studied fasting coined the term "refeeding syndrome."[13] Refeeding syndrome is a dangerous shift in the blood in which electrolytes, especially potassium, drop too low in the blood in response to a dramatic increase in insulin. One of insulin's less-appreciated effects is to push potassium into cells and out of the blood (much like what insulin does with glucose). When potassium gets too low, the heart and neurons stop working, which is rapidly lethal. This highlights the importance of breaking your fast with a meal that doesn't spike insulin; all the more reason to focus on protein and fat.

Alternatives: Overnight Fasts and Mini-Fasts

Depending on your health or where you're starting, fasting for any prolonged period of time may be the worst place to start. This is rarely a metabolic problem—our bodies are designed to be able to take prolonged breaks from food. In our experience, the people who find fasting the most challenging either are taking medications that make it difficult (exogenous insulin, sulfonylureas, etc.) or are addicted to feeling full.

Medications that increase insulin level will lower available nutrients in the blood, including glucose, fatty acids, and ketones. Remember, insulin wants to store nutrients, and it does so by either preventing them from coming into the blood from storage cells (like fatty acids from fat cells) or increasing the rate at which they enter cells (like glucose into muscle cells). Ultimately, this leaves the brain wondering what happened to all the fuel. Unlike muscle and fat cells, the brain doesn't have any significant amount of energy stored, so it's reliant on nutrients from the blood. When those nutrients start to drop, the brain signals that it's time to eat more: hunger.

Food addictions are a heavily debated topic, but compelling evidence suggests that they are real and, interestingly, that it may not be that a person is addicted to a specific food (such as sugar), but rather addicted to feeling full.[14] This can make fasting very uncomfortable, and it's all the more reason to start small.

There are two simple approaches you can focus on:

1. **Don't eat anything after dinner each evening so you can have about 12 hours of fasting each night.** Depending on your insulin resistance and what you eat, if you eat dinner around 6 p.m., it will likely take insulin 3 to 4 hours to return to normal fasting levels. That gives your body about 8 hours of resetting your insulin sensitivity as insulin remains low for much of the rest of the night.

2. **Rely on mini-fasts—eating three meals during the day, but nothing in between the meals.** Another way of describing this could be "no-snack fasts." Snacking is the antithesis of fasting and it's a habit that needs to be broken. Getting a solid 4 to 5 hours between meals is a great first step to training your body to grow accustomed to fasting.

Diana on Fasting

After practicing fasting for a few years, if I were to sum up my feelings about it in one word, that word would be *empowering*. Having the discipline to intentionally abstain from food, and quickly reap the benefits, takes you off the frantic hamster wheel where you feel like you're constantly running toward the next meal. With fasting, *you* are in control, not your hunger pangs or cravings. This freedom and power should not be underestimated.

Still, I can vividly remember my initial terror at the thought of skipping a meal. *Not eat? Gasp! That sounds like a special form of torture! Who in their right mind would voluntarily go hours or days without food?!* The first thing to note is that when your diet is primarily composed of carbohydrates, it is much more painful to skip meals. That's due to your body being in sugar-burning mode, rather than fat-burning mode (learn all about this in *Why We Get Sick*). By shifting over to a fat-fueled diet, your body will be much more comfortable in a fasted state.

To develop your own fasting practice, you can take baby steps. Start with mini-fasts, which can be a very powerful—and easy—habit to develop. Then, start skipping some meals and see how it feels. For me, refraining from food overnight and until midday or early afternoon is a comfortable, daily way to utilize the power of fasting. The next step might be to refrain from food for a full day or longer. Most weeks I like to fast from Sunday evening (after our weekly steak dinner!) until Monday dinner.

Feeling differently about fasting yet? I can't wait for you to find as much enjoyment and empowerment in it as I do!

Fasting for Women: Additional Concerns

Men and women have different levels of several hormones, including those outside the realm of sex hormones. Fasting can change hormones involved with hunger (leptin, ghrelin, etc.) and nutrient metabolism (insulin, glucagon, etc.). Generally, these results are positive, but there is one study that hints that the benefits may not be equal.

A 2005 study in normal-weight women and men tested alternate-day fasting for three weeks.[15] While the men had an improvement in insulin sensitivity, the women had no improvement. However, a more recent 6-month study in overweight/obese women found that intermittent (5-2) fasting improved every marker of metabolic health, insulin sensitivity included.[16] A follow-up study by this same research group once again studied fasting in overweight women, but this time they prescribed a particular diet.[17] Rather than just fasting, they had two protocols: one low-carbohydrate *and* low-calorie, and the other low-carbohydrate but *unlimited* calories. Both of these fasting regimens improved insulin sensitivity as well as myriad metabolic markers to a greater degree than the control diet.

Beyond the metabolic, there is some concern that fasting may compromise fertility in women. This concern isn't entirely baseless, insofar as females have a particular reliance on body fat for normal fertility. Fat releases hormones, such as leptin, that are necessary to signal to the brain to activate the release of sex hormones from the ovaries. However, short of running out of fat, fasting appears to have no negative effect on sex hormone production or fertility in humans. In fact, evidence suggests the opposite. In women with polycystic ovary syndrome (PCOS), fasting appears to help improve sex hormones, lowering testosterone and increasing estrogens to help return a healthy ovarian cycle.[18]

Reverse, Prevent, Maintain: Our Recommendations for Fasting

Where you are metabolically sheds light on where to start. It's unfortunate but true that those who need fasting the least have the easiest time with it, and those that struggle with fasting likely need it the most. See Diana's tips for starting a fasting practice on the previous page.

> **MAINTAIN:** If you're already insulin sensitive and seek to maintain your status, longer fasts (18+ hours) should be almost a daily occurrence, or at least three times per week. You could also benefit from a full 24-hour fast weekly.
>
> **PREVENT:** If you're sliding into insulin resistance or recently coming out of it, fasting might be a struggle. If not, aim for the same guidelines outlined in "Maintain." If it's hard for you, aim for the guidelines outlined in "Reverse."
>
> **REVERSE:** If you're insulin resistant, the chronically elevated insulin will make it harder to rely on your body fat for fuel (remember, insulin stops fat cells from breaking down fat to be burned by the body). Start with a 12-hour fast each day (i.e., no snacking after dinner) and avoid snacking between meals. This modest beginning will bear fruit later.

Prioritize Protein

When it comes to insulin resistance and metabolic health, what you eat can be the culprit or the cure. Of all the interventions you can undertake to reverse or prevent insulin resistance, diet will bring the biggest change—which means that your health is very much under your control.

By focusing on getting the right intake of the three macronutrients—protein, fat, and carbohydrates—we can see the beginnings of a dietary plan to put into action. While many of us get the balance wrong, when you're armed with the knowledge of *what to eat* and *why*—those macronutrients' function in our diet—actually doing it might become a lot easier. So over the next three chapters, we'll look at the three main strategies: prioritize protein, don't fear fat, and control carbohydrates.

Why We Prioritize Protein

Protein is a building block of life, so it should be no surprise that many amino acids (molecules that combine to form proteins—or the building blocks of the building blocks) are essential to humans—we must eat them to survive. When the human body lacks protein, bad things happen: muscle and bone wasting, anemia, and (on the extreme end) stunted growth, liver failure, and more. Many of us don't eat enough protein. Inasmuch as most people with insulin resistance are more mature in years, protein is even more relevant—the older we get, the harder it is for us to digest and use the protein we eat.[1]

So protein is important for health. Eating it also gives you sustained energy. However, some clinicians, scientists, and members of the general public within the "low-carb community" are wary of protein because it elicits an insulin response (or, actually, the amino acid does). While this can happen, the context is important—and often overlooked. That context is glucose.

Your health is very much under your control.

When you eat protein either with carbohydrates or when your blood glucose is elevated, the amino acids from the protein will amplify the normal glucose-induced insulin response. (This might be why carbohydrates and protein very, very rarely come together in nature.) However, when protein is consumed without carbohydrates, either alone or (as *does* occur in nature) with fat, the insulin secretion is substantially reduced.[2] Interestingly, in addition to a much smaller insulin release, the pancreas also releases a much larger amount of glucagon—insulin's opposite. Whereas insulin seeks to store energy, glucagon wants to burn it. As a result, in such a metabolic state, the insulin-to-glucagon ratio actually stays pretty steady despite the protein-induced insulin bump. And frankly, this is an instance when we want insulin increased—not only does the insulin help our cells take in the amino acids but it also protects the proteins in the muscles from being broken down.

How Much Protein?

The idea that an insulin-smart diet needs to be low in protein is simply incorrect. Some of this sentiment is borne from the early implementation of ketogenic diets in children to control epilepsy, where any insulin spike, and the potential for inhibiting ketogenesis, is a concern. However, outside of this narrow therapeutic instance, the vast majority of clinical studies in humans exploring low-carbohydrate or ketogenic diets have had protein levels anywhere from 20% to 30% of total calories.

In scientific circles, one of the most popular studies ever published on the metabolic effects of ketogenic diets had what many would consider to be too much protein (but, spoiler alert, we do not). In 2009, scientists at the University of Connecticut and other institutions recruited subjects to participate in a perfectly controlled 12-week study.[3] Every scrap of food was accounted for by directly feeding every subject for each meal every day. While the calories were identical across the groups, the composition of the diet varied greatly. One group had a diet that was designed to mimic the standard American diet (i.e., relatively low in fat and high in carbohydrate). The ketogenic group had the opposite diet (i.e., low carbohydrate and high fat). Importantly, while protein constituted 28% of calories in the ketogenic diet group (vs. 20% in the low-fat group), those subjects had an increase in insulin sensitivity that was dramatically better than the high-carbohydrate group. Furthermore, any insulin bump from the dietary protein was so modest that it didn't prevent ketogenesis.

To get adequate protein, aim for at least 1.5 grams (g) of protein daily per kilogram (kg) of your *ideal* body weight. If you weigh 200 pounds (90 kg) but know you should weigh around 150 pounds (68 kg), try to get a minimum of 102 g (1.5 × 68) of protein daily (unless you're fasting). In the meal plans in this book, protein makes up 30% of the daily caloric intake.

What Kind of Protein?

Our ancestors would have obtained virtually all their dietary protein from animal sources, whether from meat, seafood, eggs, or dairy. In their native state, plants are generally too deficient in protein to represent a meaningful source (some nuts are exceptions). Some plant-based proteins, like tofu and tempeh, do have good amounts of protein—and we'll talk more about those shortly. However, nowadays we have created new protein-rich foods from plant sources—like peas and pumpkin seeds—that our ancestors wouldn't recognize in their new forms. While these modern proteins are a wonder of technology, they have considerations.

First, plants are naturally very low in proteins, which means that in order to get enough protein from peas, for example, you need to concentrate the protein by collecting amino acids from a *lot* of them—in a serving of peas (~200 grams), only about 2% of it will be protein. In concentrating the protein, other molecules get concentrated along with it.

As noted, proteins are made up of amino acids, and some of these amino acids are considered "essential"—meaning we must eat them—while others can be made in the body, and are thus termed "nonessential." The list of essential amino acids isn't long; there are nine of them: histidine, isoleucine, leucine (the most important for muscle growth), lysine, methionine, phenylalanine, threonine, tryptophan, and valine.

Animal proteins contain all essential amino acids. Moreover, they come in a form that is readily usable—our bodies absorb animal proteins very well. Unfortunately, despite their popularity, plant proteins aren't quite as clear-cut.[4] You would need to eat a wide variety of plants to ensure you're getting all the essential amino acids. And with the newer plant-based proteins, there are two other considerations, which both have to do with unwanted guests.

> **Animal proteins contain all essential amino acids. Moreover, they come in a form that is readily usable . . . Plant proteins aren't quite as clear-cut.**

The first category of unwanted guests is antinutrients. These nutrient villains are a class of molecules that work against the body digesting and absorbing nutrients. Lectins,[5] phytates,[6] tannins,[7] and more naturally occur in plants and collectively compromise the absorption of several minerals, such as zinc, iron, and magnesium. This is one of the main reasons so many plants around the world are inedible. We've selectively bred food plants to have very few of these antinutrients. That is, until we concentrate them.

The second category of unwanted guests is more harmful minerals, such as lead and arsenic (called "heavy metals" due to their atomic mass). These metal minerals can accumulate in our cells and result in oxidative stress and other harmful changes. Plants naturally pull in metals from the soil, albeit to a very low degree. But, once again, when we concentrate the plant matter to get to the protein, we increase the risk of getting potentially harmful levels of antinutrients and metals.[8]

Of course, humans have been getting protein from plants for generations, so if plant proteins have the potential for such harm, why have we persisted? It could be that modern technology is working against us. Tofu is a good example. Traditionally, tofu, derived from soybean curd, would be fermented. Fermentation diminishes antinutrients, subsequently enhancing the overall digestibility and bioavailability of minerals and amino acids.[9] Fermenting can also reduce the amount of metals.[10] (Just two of the many wonders of fermentation, which we'll come back to later in this chapter!)

Animal proteins give you all of the essential amino acids you need. If you are obtaining most of your dietary protein from plants, consider seeking fermented sources to help ensure you're getting more of what you want from the food (protein), and less of what you don't want (antinutrients and heavy metals).

With all this in mind, here's a short list of ideal protein sources and their nutritional breakdown, based on a conventional serving size of 4 ounces (115 g):

Insulin-Friendly Protein (4 oz / 115 g)	Fats (g)	Net Carbs (g)	Protein (g)
Ground beef (80/20)	23	0	20
Rib-eye steak	25	0	27
Bacon	51	0	13
Pork chop	18	0	30
Chicken thigh	20	0	17
Chicken breast	1	0	26
Salmon	15	0	23
Ground lamb	27	0	19
Large egg	5	0.5	6
Tofu	3	2	7
Tempeh	9	9	15
Pumpkin seeds	42	4	32
Peanut butter	50	14	25

A final consideration is protein's natural companion—fat. As noted, animal-sourced proteins also come with fat. In our misguided fear of fat, we have pulled the protein away from fat, and this is a mistake for two reasons.

First is the matter of digestion. When we teach and think about protein digestion, we tend to compartmentalize its process and only discuss the proteolytic enzymes—those that are specifically designed to break apart the bonds between amino acids. Proteolysis happens because without it, proteins are much too big to move through the intestines and be absorbed.

Interestingly, however, these protein-specific enzymes don't act in isolation. When fat is consumed, it wants to ball together, which prevents the fat-specific digestive enzymes from pulling off individual fat molecules. The intestines have a way to account for this—bile. Bile, which is produced in the liver and stored in the gallbladder, is squeezed into the intestines when we eat fat, and the bile pulls the fat blobs apart so that the digestive enzymes can do their job. But bile isn't just a player in fat metabolism; bile facilitates the proteolytic enzymes as well, accelerating protein digestion by allowing the amino acid bonds to be split.[11] However, dietary protein doesn't have the same bile-releasing effect that dietary fat does. In other words, to ensure you fully digest protein, a little fat goes a long way.

And after digestion, we want the proteins to help us build and maintain muscle. But once again, proteins aren't meant to do this alone. In a study of exercising college-aged males, research subjects were given a load of protein from egg whites or a whole egg—the egg white plus yolk. The whole egg, yolk and all, elicited far greater muscle growth than the whites alone.[12] While this might sound surprising, it makes sense when we consider that proteins help build the bulk of the muscle cell, while fats are a primary component of the muscle cell wall. So if the muscle cell is growing, you need enough fats to keep the cell membrane intact to accommodate that growth.

However, in stating all this, we don't mean to do dietary fat a disservice by making it sound like it's simply protein's sidekick—fat is a macronutrient hero in its own right, and we'll look at why in the next chapter.

If you are obtaining most of your dietary protein from plants, consider seeking fermented sources to help ensure you're getting more of what you want from the food (protein), and less of what you don't want (antinutrients and heavy metals).

Ben on BCAAs

Within the family of essential amino acids are the three musketeers of muscle protein—leucine, isoleucine, and valine—the branched-chain amino acids (BCAAs), so called due to their chemical structure. Because these are the amino acids most enriched in muscle proteins, they're very popular among those who want to grow and maintain muscle mass (BCAAs are found in almost every workout supplement). However, there has been growing concern that BCAAs might contribute to insulin resistance.

First, there is evidence that people with insulin resistance have higher circulating BCAA levels in the blood—but this is a correlational (i.e., coincidental) finding, which of course does not establish causation. Insulin protects muscle proteins by inhibiting their breakdown, helping the muscle keep its hard-earned protein and mass. However, as the muscle becomes insulin resistant, the loss of insulin's protective effect can lead to greater muscle protein breakdown. Because the BCAAs are so enriched in muscle, they are subsequently "leaked" more readily out of the diminishing muscle and into the blood. Thus, in this paradigm, far from *causing* insulin resistance, elevated BCAAs might be a *consequence* of it.

This model is challenged, though. There is some causal evidence that adds to the growing anti-BCAA sentiment and is admittedly harder to overlook. When people with type 2 diabetes eat a diet low in BCAAs, insulin sensitivity improves, at least in the short term.[1] That doesn't prove that BCAAs *cause* insulin resistance. The closest evidence for that is in rodent studies. Even then, the evidence is conflicted. While some studies show that all three BCAAs can exacerbate insulin resistance in a rodent model of type 2 diabetes (though not in healthy rodents), leucine alone, which is the amino acid that matters most for muscle growth, improves insulin sensitivity in muscle and the liver.[2] However, others have noted that when muscle cells are exposed to normal levels of BCAAs, as opposed to the "super-physiological" doses often used in animal studies, there is no issue with insulin resistance.[3] Personally, I do not believe there is any reason to fear amino acids or restrict them in any way.

1 Karusheva, Y., et al. *Short-term dietary reduction of branched-chain amino acids reduces meal-induced insulin secretion and modifies microbiome composition in type 2 diabetes: a randomized controlled crossover trial.* Am J Clin Nutr, 2019. **110**(5): p. 1098-107.

2 Zeanandin, G., et al. *Differential effect of long-term leucine supplementation on skeletal muscle and adipose tissue in old rats: an insulin signaling pathway approach.* Age (Dordr), 2012. **34**(2): p. 371-87.

3 Rivera, M. E., C. N. Rivera, and R. A. Vaughan. *Branched-chain amino acids at supraphysiological but not physiological levels reduce myotube insulin sensitivity.* Diabetes Metab Res Rev, 2022. **38**(2): p. e3490; Rivera, M. E., C. N. Rivera, and R. A. Vaughan. *Excess branched-chain amino acids alter myotube metabolism and substrate preference which is worsened by concurrent insulin resistance.* Endocrine, 2022. **76**(1): p. 18-28.

Don't Fear Fat

We mean it—quit being so afraid of dietary fat. If you were around in the '90s, then this might be a tough sell, but bear with us. The notion that *fat makes you fat* has lived on way past its expiration date. Far from being the metabolic villain we've heard about for the past 50 years, dietary fat is a healthy and even necessary component of the human diet. Even more, it's the most benign of the macronutrients when it comes to insulin (see the figure below), which makes it a smart addition to a dietary plan that seeks to improve insulin resistance.

But this is a hard lesson to learn—it requires unlearning decades of anti-fat messaging. Let us help with some of that.

The fear of dietary fat was borne from a fear of heart disease (and sometime later this progressed to encompass obesity, diabetes, cancer, and every other chronic disease). As happens so often, these conclusions were based on correlational studies, which tended to suggest that eating saturated fat can increase LDL cholesterol, and LDL cholesterol is associated with heart disease. Unfortunately, this ideology took hold so firmly that scientists in the

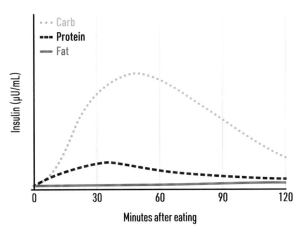

Notes from Ben's Lab

Dietary fat and its metabolic consequences is a topic I'm very familiar with. The primary focus of my post-doctoral fellowship was to study the effects of a particular immune pathway in causing insulin resistance in various cell types. To activate this pathway, we treated cells directly with certain fats or infused certain types of fat mixtures directly into the blood of research animals. Following the fat incubation or infusion, we'd test the cells' or animals' responsiveness to insulin and invariably find a reduced response—the fat caused insulin resistance. This fortified my own belief that fat, particularly saturated fat, was a cause of insulin resistance.

However, even at the time, I had a nagging doubt that what I was seeing was an artifact of the experimental model, and not a true physiological finding: treating cells with fats or directly infusing fats intravenously is not the same as *eating* fat. (Of course, it obviously isn't, but you'd be surprised at how often these kinds of ideas are conflated.)

At the same time as I was causing insulin resistance with fat incubations (in cells) and infusions (in rodents), I was seeing evidence that chronic elevations in insulin can cause insulin resistance. I knew enough at the time to realize that fat has very little or no effect on insulin—this paradox prompted me to look into *human* clinical studies that altered macronutrients (e.g., low-carbohydrate versus low-fat diets). When I learned that low-carbohydrate diets that were high in fat, even saturated fat, improved insulin resistance to a greater degree than low-fat, high-carbohydrate diets, I saw the problem with my fat-based studies—I was ignoring the physiology of fat digestion and absorption and fat metabolism in cells. Understanding those processes will help you understand why we're making such a strong case for healthy fats as part of an insulin-sensitizing lifestyle.

mid-1900s (when these ideas came to life) who had contrary evidence often simply elected to not share their findings for fear of swift and career-ending retribution.[1] (Unfortunately, the professional pressure to toe the line is still very much alive. As a scientist who has elected to challenge dietary dogma, Ben can attest to the temptation to "keep your head down" due to professional, and sometimes personal, attacks.)

The Case for Fat

When we eat fat, after it is digested (thanks, bile!) and absorbed, the fats are transported as triglycerides on chylomicrons, which are large lipoproteins. Most of the fats are taken to the liver, though some are deposited in tissues on the way there. Once in the liver, fat can be repackaged and sent back out into the body on the triglyceride-rich lipoproteins (very-low-density and low-density lipoproteins; VLDL and LDL). To make the case in favor of fat, there are several important points to consider.

The first helpful point is that the fat we eat is *not* the fat that circulates in our blood. This phenomenon is emphasized well in a study published in 2008. Over a 12-week period, study subjects were fed either a low-fat or a high-fat diet (with inverse levels of carbohydrates in each), with the high-fat diet containing over three times more saturated fat than the low-fat diet (all matched for total calories).[2] Despite this threefold greater consumption of saturated fats in the diet, the actual amount of saturated fats in the blood of those subjects was *lower* than for those in the low-fat group!

There are two explanations for this. First, cells, especially liver cells, have the unique ability to alter the chemical nature of fat molecules to suit the cells' needs. The liver is a critical way station in this process because the very nature of the fats can be altered in this step. Specifically, cells can *desaturate* saturated fats, turning a saturated fat into a monounsaturated fat. In fact, the most common product of this process is oleate—the fat most commonly found in olive oil. Not only does this mean that blood saturated fats are reduced but also that the most common fat in our fat cells isn't palmitate (the most commonly consumed fat—a saturated fat), but rather oleate! It's not even close, actually—a fat cell has on average twice as much fat stored as oleate compared with palmitate,[3] even though we eat much more palmitate than oleate.

The next explanation for how eating saturated fat (in the context of a low-carbohydrate diet) can lower circulating levels of saturated fat is an overlooked aspect of insulin. Insulin is the metabolic master hormone and the liver is one of its favorite targets. When insulin is elevated, the liver is determined to store energy. Fats can store more energy in the body than glucose—by well over 100 times. To help insulin promote an energy storage state in the body, the liver aggressively pulls in glucose and turns it into fat, a process known as *de novo lipogenesis*. The product of this fat-making process is palmitate! This is why a person could avoid all saturated fats completely but, by eating insulin-spiking carbohydrates, still have higher circulating saturated fat levels than someone eating loads of saturated fats but avoiding insulin-spiking foods.

This is a great time to mention another human study that sought to understand the role of saturated fats in health and disease. One of the most famous diets ever is a plan created to help reduce heart disease by lowering blood pressure—the DASH (dietary approaches to stop hypertension) diet. This diet is based on a few pivotal pillars: eat fruits and vegetables, reduce salt, avoid excess sugar, and eat low-fat foods. The positive results from this diet in lowering blood pressure have reinforced the call to avoid salt and fat, in particular. However, some scientists just don't know when to quit, and in 2016, a research group in California asked: *What would happen if we replaced all the low-fat foods with high-fat foods?* This meant no more low-fat dairy or lean meat or no butter—it was a fatty-food bonanza. Over the course of the study, the high-fat DASH group ended up eating almost twice the amount of total fat and twice the amount of saturated fat compared with the classic DASH diet group.[4] Despite this seemingly catastrophic diet, the high-fat DASH diet actually outperformed the low-fat version, resulting in a significant reduction in triglycerides (the primary circulating form of fats) and the triglyceride:HDL ratio, a commonly used metric of insulin resistance. Importantly, in addition to improving blood lipids *better* than its low-fat competitor, the high-fat DASH diet also lowered blood pressure just as much.

The second helpful point in shifting the blame away from saturated fats is that lipoproteins are not bad. Remember, the potential of increasing LDL was originally the primary reason to avoid saturated fat. As flawed as this logic is, the tragedy is made worse by completely overlooking LDL's positive role. Yes, LDL is a transport mechanism to move fats (in the form of triglycerides and cholesterol) around the body, but it's also a critical component of the immune system. To put this in perspective, we need to introduce a villain: lipopolysaccharides (LPS).

LPS are molecules that exist on the membranes of a massive family of bacteria, and these membrane fragments are everywhere; LPS is found in the food we eat, the water we drink, and even, in some instances, the air we breathe.[5] However it gets in, LPS activates potent immune and inflammatory signals in cells throughout the body. To help prevent it from stimulating too much inflammation, we want to remove the invader as quickly as possible. LDL is unique in that it can neutralize LPS by binding to it. Not only does this prevent LPS from activating inflammatory processes but it also acts as an escort mechanism. Once bound, LDL won't let go until it passes LPS into the liver, at which point the liver promptly moves it into the bile duct, where it eventually ends up in the intestines. At this point, the battle is won. LPS meets an inglorious ending. This anti-LPS and immune-protective effect of LDL cholesterol very much explains why people with higher LDL levels are significantly less likely to experience severe infections.[6]

In a broader sense beyond immunity, the protective effects of LDL cholesterol are even more relevant. We've known for decades that people with higher cholesterol levels live longer than people with lower cholesterol. This is a persistent finding, with groups from the US to China coming to similar conclusions.[7]

To put a finer and final point on defending dietary fat, it's been shown to explicitly help various neurological conditions,[8] fertility,[9] and more.[10] Clearly, there's more to fat than most of us appreciate.

What Kind of Fat?

Throughout this discussion on dietary fat, you might have noticed a theme suggesting the types of fats we should focus on. In general, don't fear natural fats, namely those that come from animals or fatty fruits, like coconuts, avocados, or olives. However, you should fear unnatural fats— those that come from refined seed oils, commonly referred to as "vegetable oils." Don't let that clever marketing fool you—there's nothing "vegetable" about "vegetable oil" (it just sounds better than "refined seed oils").

Naturally saturated fats are healthy partly because they're so stable. When fats have several unsaturated carbon bonds, they are understandably called polyunsaturated fats. These fats abound in refined seed oils, and they are the fats we've been told to eat for decades now because they may have an effect on lowering cholesterol. Unfortunately, they are remarkably harmful. Each of the unsaturated bonds increases the potential for the fat to become a peroxide—these are basically the unholy offspring of the union between oxidative stress and a fat. Once created, peroxides have the potential to damage everything, including mitochondria, cell membranes, and even DNA.[11] Saturated fats, however, experience none of this—their saturated structures means they're highly resistant to the pathogenic process of peroxidation.

At the height of the anti-fat wars (1968–1973), a group in the US conducted a study that couldn't be done in the modern era. People living in institutions were placed on two diets differing in the composition of fat type: one group eating more saturated fats, and the other more polyunsaturated fats. After following these diets for several years, researchers paid scrupulous attention to the health of the study subjects. The initial findings simply reported that

> Don't fear natural fats, namely those that come from animals or fatty fruits, like coconuts, avocados, or olives. However, you should fear unnatural fats—those that come from refined seed oils, commonly referred to as "vegetable oils."

the polyunsaturated fat diet resulted in lower blood cholesterol. However, a re-analysis of the data decades later revealed that the lower cholesterol offered no health benefit, and in fact, for each 30 mg/dL reduction in cholesterol, mortality increased by 22%![12] To make matters even worse (for the polyunsaturated fat eaters), there was no difference in heart disease rates between the groups.

A parallel study was conducted on the other side of the world around this same time (1966–1973).[13] Like the US study, the Australian study similarly attempted to hide its results (you can never keep good data down!) . . . and for good reason. This time, it was even more difficult to reconcile with the idea that saturated fats are bad. After re-analyzing the original data, the authors concluded that substituting polyunsaturated fats for saturated fats "increased the rates of death from all causes, coronary heart disease, and cardiovascular disease."

These are *the* best studies ever published on the topic, and if there were ever evidence that saturated fats caused health problems over a long enough term to detect disease, these studies would have revealed it. Far from the authors' original intentions of using these studies to demonize saturated fats, it found them innocent of all charges.

A final comment clarification on why refined seed oils should be avoided has to do with the fat cell itself. The fat that circulates in our blood generally becomes the fat that is stored in our fat cells. Of course, this doesn't hold entirely true with regard to saturated fats, as noted earlier, insofar as they're often desaturated and further altered. However, the primary fat in refined seed oils is the polyunsaturated fat linoleic acid. This fat does get enriched in fat cells,[14] but it doesn't often remain as an innocent fat. Remember, the more unsaturated the fat, the greater the potential for it to become a peroxide. As we have covered, the fat cell is the likely point of origin when it comes to insulin resistance in the body—it's the first domino to fall, bumping into other tissues, like muscle, liver, and more, to spread insulin resistance throughout the body. Several noxious stimuli can turn a good fat cell bad, but an important one is the molecule that is formed from the peroxidation of the linoleic acid. As this molecule accumulates, it forces fat cells to grow through hypertrophy (which we first explored in chapter 1—see page 22).

By now, you may understandably think I'm declaring war on all polyunsaturated fats. Not so! Technically, I'm urging caution surrounding omega-6 polyunsaturated fats and, more specifically, linoleic acid. However, omega-3 fats, which are also polyunsaturated, are resistant to these pathological changes[15] and have a couple of noteworthy benefits that are overlooked.

Everybody touts the apparent benefits of omega-3 fats in heart disease based on correlational studies (which as you now know should be viewed with some skepticism). However, better-controlled studies have found more novel results. Did you know that omega-3 fats can help build muscle? We are so quick to only promote protein as the macronutrient of muscle building, but even taken in the absence of protein entirely, omega-3 fats have been shown to enhance muscle building.[16] At the same time, omega-3 fats make fat cells "run hotter"! They may increase the metabolic rate in fat cells,[17] which would help control fat cell growth. That's a neat idea, isn't it—fat helping fat cells burn more fat!

In the end, don't be so afraid of fat—unless it's from a refined seed oil. If the fat is derived from fats we have been eating for millennia, namely fruit fats and animal fats, enjoy liberally. Some nut oils, such as macadamia nut, are also fine.

> There is so much enjoyment and satisfaction to be found in increasing the amount of wholesome fat in your diet. Food that contains fat typically tastes amazing (think butter, cheese, and red meats). Fueling up on fat also keeps you full longer.

There is so much enjoyment and satisfaction to be found in increasing the amount of wholesome fat in your diet. Food that contains fat typically tastes amazing (think butter, cheese, and red meats). Fueling up on fat also keeps you full longer. Gone are the energy surges and crashes with pesky hunger pangs that interrupt your day. You're able to view food as the fuel source that it is, with a job to power your body, rather than a constantly required resource.

5

Control Carbohydrates

We've said it before and we'll say it again: a primary cause of insulin resistance is chronically elevated insulin. Thus, a highly effective way to start improving is to allow your insulin to be low. With this view, it's easy to see why dietary carbohydrates need to be put in their place. Carbohydrates represent the primary source of calories in the modern diet, but putting them in last place is the better position. Unfortunately, a diet that contains too much carbohydrates can double a person's fasting insulin in just a week.[1] *Why We Get Sick* highlighted dozens of articles that outline the results of clinical studies on restricting carbohydrates. A nice way to summarize the impact of these myriad studies is to mention this: the evidence is so overwhelming that even the American Diabetes Association announced that "most evidence" supports carbohydrate restriction for improving type 2 diabetes (i.e., insulin resistance).[2]

Importantly, the insulin-sensitizing benefit of carbohydrate restriction is at least as good as, and often better than, calorie restriction.[3] This is meaningful. As discussed in chapter 2, simply eating less (or not eating at all) can lower insulin and improve insulin resistance. However, eating less will often drive hunger, which makes sticking with a dietary plan very challenging. But providing a mechanism whereby insulin drops and hunger is kept in control, as is the case with a carbohydrate-controlled diet, there's a clear path forward.

Independent of the effect on insulin, one reason to bump carbohydrates out of first place in the diet is because they *aren't needed*. Don't misunderstand—this is not to say you should never eat carbohydrates—they can be a perfectly fine part of an insulin-sensitizing dietary plan. However, they *literally* are not needed for human survival or thriving. The Food and Nutrition Board of the US Institute of Medicine (now the National Academy of Medicine) stated: "The lower limit of dietary carbohydrate compatible with life apparently is zero, provided that adequate amounts of protein and fat are consumed."[4]

Glucose, the nutrient that flows in the blood, *is* necessary, but blood glucose is *not* dietary carbohydrate. Yes, dietary carbohydrates are digested into glucose that enters the blood and is then used as a fuel, thus the glucose we eat is *one* source of blood glucose. But our liver is capable of *making* glucose on its own, through a process known as gluconeogenesis. Whatever need the body has for glucose—for example, by the brain or red blood cells—is met by the liver. In a fascinating process of metabolic alchemy, the liver is able to convert muscle-derived lactate into glucose.

That's right—lactate, the dreaded molecule that so many erroneously claim makes muscles sore, though it does no such thing! Far from being a villain, lactate is a vehicle for recycling potential chemical energy to keep glucose levels normal. This is why a person can fast, eating no calories whatsoever, and retain a perfectly normal glucose level. If it weren't for the liver and its ability to recycle nutrients into glucose, we'd all become hypoglycemic after a day of fasting and die shortly after.

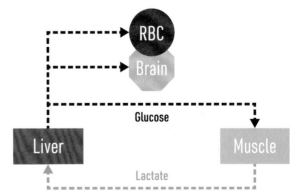

When we talk about controlling carbs, there are three considerations: what kind, when, and how much.

Uric Acid and Inflammation

Recently, a new potential contributor to insulin resistance has come on the scene that deserves some attention: uric acid. Uric acid is produced in several reactions in the body, but the most common in the modern diet is through the metabolism of fructose. Every molecule of fructose that gets used for energy produces a molecule of uric acid. As you probably know, most of us eat a lot of sugar, which is half fructose—and those of us who drink fruit juice are drinking straight fructose. So we metabolize a lot of fructose, and subsequently get a lot of uric acid.

Classically, the most obvious concern with uric acid was gout, but it very clearly has an effect on insulin resistance. When cells are incubated with uric acid, they become insulin resistant. When insulin-resistant rodents and humans are treated with drugs that inhibit uric acid, they become insulin sensitive. That said, we won't focus too much on uric acid because it likely acts *through inflammation*.[1] In other words, if you remove the inflammation from the equation, uric acid may not affect insulin resistance.

Unfortunately, there is little we can do regarding inflammation—it's simply too slippery and too vague. There's no doubt that inflammation matters (especially in light of the overfat fat cells we discussed in chapter 1). But if a person has an autoimmune disease, for instance, and experiences higher levels of inflammatory proteins, insulin resistance will follow the ebb and flow of the disease. Despite this, uric acid does promote inflammation, and thus is relevant in any strategy to control inflammation—less dietary fructose will lead to reduced uric acid levels, which will ease the pressure on inflammation.

What Kind of Carbs?

Our simple (and memorable, we hope) rule is that if the carbohydrates come in a bag or a box with a barcode, avoid or eat sparingly. This is, of course, a bit simplistic, but it can act as a guide. A baked potato, for example, will be much better than French fries or potato chips—this has to do with the degree to which the carbohydrate is processed.

Think of carbohydrates as having "degrees of refinement"—how many times the item has been altered. For example, apple juice goes through two degrees of refinement (crushing and filtering), so it will have a far greater glucose-insulin impact than an apple. Similarly, coarse wheat will have a more modest glucose-insulin effect compared with bread because the latter has gone through several degrees of refinement (milled, bleached, fortified, baked, etc.). An interesting study scrutinized the effects of these kinds of refinements to food in an experiment with lab animals, where all variables can be controlled. These animals were fed two diets that differed only in the degree of refinement—whole pellets versus powdered meal. Again, the diets were exactly the same in every nutrient. In addition to being more inclined to overeat, the animals that were fed the powdered version of the diets gained over twice the amount of fat and had significantly higher insulin and glucose levels.[5]

Another fascinating consideration to dietary carbohydrates is fermentation. A common "degree of refinement" in carbohydrate foods is adding chemicals to preserve them and prevent spoiling. Add to this our ability to refrigerate foods as well, which slows the process of decay, and we effectively prevent little bacteria from doing what they'd like with carbohydrates . . . namely, eat them, through the process of fermentation, which we touched on briefly earlier in this chapter and bears a closer look now.

Fermentation involves bacteria digesting dietary carbohydrates (fructose, lactose, glucose, etc.) and producing very short fatty acids (giving a slightly tart taste), carbon dioxide (giving a drink some bubbles or food some air pockets), and, possibly, alcohol (ranging from trace amounts to high, depending on the nature and length of ferment). The chemical products are interesting and even metabolically valuable, but it's what's lost, not gained, in the process of fermenting that may be particularly relevant in exploring the insulin-sensitizing benefits of fermented food.

Bacteria have a sweet tooth—they eat only carbohydrates (starches and sugars) from food items in fermentation, leaving untouched any proteins and fats. As a result, bacteria bear some of the metabolic burden for us, leaving behind a foodstuff that has a much smaller impact on glucose and insulin.[6] So we have two pronounced insulin-sensitizing benefits when we consume a fermented food: we consume less starch than in the nonfermented version, and we ingest beneficial bacteria that can act as probiotics in our intestines.

In general, minimal processing is ideal with carbohydrate foods, but some processing is good. A baked potato is a great example. When we bake a potato (a degree of refinement), we make the starch in the potato much more digestible—baking foods was one of humans' earliest technological breakthroughs regarding

Ben's Favorite Fermented Food

Because this is really the only place for me to mention it, I am compelled to bring up one of my favorite fermented foods: apple cider vinegar! You may not even know that apple cider vinegar is a fermented food. Basically, once you start fermenting something in water, it will go through a fermenting journey. At first, the bacteria will eat the sugars and produce alcohol. But if the fermentation continues, the bacteria further convert the alcohol into acetic acid—the key molecule in vinegar. In fact, acetic acid is actually a fat molecule—it's the shortest (and most tart!) of all fats. But don't underestimate it due to its minuscule molecular structure, because it's actually a metabolic heavyweight. Acetic acid has myriad metabolic effects, including stimulating mitochondrial biogenesis and increasing the metabolic rate in fat cells.[1] It also increases insulin sensitivity, which is something we can leverage.

While drinking a little apple cider vinegar prior to a starchy meal can help blunt the glucose and insulin effect of that meal,[2] the benefits aren't limited to a narrow time window. Even taking 2 tablespoons of raw apple cider vinegar in the evening helps control glucose levels the following morning, when glucose levels tend to climb.[3] My recommendation is 2 tablespoons every morning and evening with water (I prefer it with sparkling water). Additionally, take a little before your largest carbohydrate-heavy meal. If you can test your glucose levels with a continuous glucose monitor, you'll be amazed at how effectively a preload with apple cider vinegar keeps the glucose under control.

food preparation. Of course, this starch converts into a rather large glucose load entering the blood, which elicits a robust insulin release to manage it. However, by cooling the potato after baking it, the starches in the potato convert into soluble fibers, thereby lowering the glucose load. In fact, the insulin demand from eating a baked potato is almost 40% lower if the baked potato has been cooled to room temperature before eating.[7] Thankfully, this even persists after it's been reheated!

Ultimately, the most helpful, though not always convenient, method to know whether dietary carbohydrates are going to fault or facilitate your insulin-sensitizing journey is understanding the glycemic load of the food. The glycemic load is a number that estimates how much a particular carbohydrate will raise your blood glucose. While the glycemic index measures how quickly a carbohydrate is digested into blood glucose, the glycemic load actually determines how much carbohydrate is in the food that can become glucose in the blood. In other words, glycemic load is more practical.

A watermelon is the best example. The glycemic index of watermelon is "high" at 72, which would make you think you need to avoid it. However, the glycemic load, which considers the actual amount of carbohydrate in it, is quite low at 2. Fiber-rich vegetables and fruits are a good way to enjoy carbohydrates without the insulin spike and, not surprisingly, they have very low glycemic loads. Here's a general overview:

Glycemic Load	Verdict	Examples
<15	Good	This includes leafy greens and other nonstarchy vegetables like broccoli, cauliflower, peppers, cucumbers, and more.
16-30	Be careful	This range includes berries, citrus fruits, certain less starchy vegetables like carrots and peas, and baked potatoes (remember, the glycemic load drops when it's cooled).
>30	Danger	The "danger zone" is every processed food, juices, breads, crackers, cereals, ice cream, sugary fruits like pineapples and bananas, and so many more.

When it comes to fruits and vegetables, it's best to try to balance the glycemic load with the nutrients—focus on those that are high in vitamins and minerals and low in glucose/fructose. Here are some good fruits and vegetables that meet the criteria of "control carbohydrates" (average serving size 100 g).[8] Of course, the glycemic load for any fruit or vegetable will drop considerably with fermentation.

Insulin-Friendly Fruits and Vegetables (100 g)	Fats (g)	Net Carbs (g)	Protein (g)
Cabbage	0	6	2
Cauliflower	0	6	5
Broccoli	1	7	5
Spinach	0	1	3
Romaine Lettuce	1	2	2
Bell Pepper	0	5	1
Green Beans	0	4	2
Onion	0	12	2
Blackberries	1	8	2
Raspberries	1	8	2

How Much Carbohydrate?

While the type of carbs you eat is generally more important than how much you eat, the amount does matter if you want to keep insulin under control. The plans outlined later in this book provide specific ranges built on your insulin resistance status. And, in general, the amounts suggested are probably going to be less than what you're used to if you've been eating a typical Western diet. It is time to rethink your relationship with carbs.

We get it. Breakups are tough, especially when deep down you'd rather stay together. We're not going to lie to you and say that carbs are unpleasant and your taste buds are better off without them. The truth is that carbs and sugar taste fantastic to us—and in general the more refined, the better tasting. This is partly due to the fact that there are actual chemical reactions taking place in the pleasure centers in your brain that "reward" you for eating carbs.[9]

Why We Count Net Carbs, Not Total Carbs

There are some macronutrient mathematics that are uniquely relevant to dietary carbohydrates. For reasons that elude common sense, dietary fiber, which offers no caloric value to the body, is considered a carbohydrate like any other. This means that if a food product has 10 grams of sugar and 10 grams of soluble fiber, the carbohydrate count will be listed as 20 grams. But when it comes to our intestines and the enzymes that digest carbohydrates into their simplest parts, the body can do nothing with dietary fiber, so those grams should not be counted.

The idea that not all dietary carbohydrates are created equal is encompassed in the term "net carbs." The simple formula is that you subtract the amount of dietary fiber from the total listed dietary carbohydrate.

In the meal plans outlined later, the suggested amounts of dietary carbohydrates are net carbs. There's no reason to include dietary fiber in your daily carb count if it has no effect on glucose and insulin.

The great news is that you don't have to *never see them again*, it's just time for some really strong boundaries. When you feel the lure of carbs, know you can call your reliable friend, fat, who has your best interests at heart.

All silliness aside, it's worth noting the difference in what your taste buds want (simple carbs) and what your body needs (wholesome fat and protein). Learning to resist the demands of your taste buds (*most of the time*) is more than half the battle when it comes to living an insulin-sensitizing lifestyle. Lucky for us there are incredibly tasty low-and no-carb foods to love. For some examples, turn to chapter 13.

When Should I Eat Carbs?

This rule is simple: carbs come last. If you plan to include carbohydrates in a meal, just eat them at the end of your meal, after you eat the protein and fat. Doing so will significantly blunt the impact of the starches and sugars.[10]

Another important timing consideration is exercise, which we'll discuss in the next chapter. There seems to be a cultural obsession with the idea that we must eat carbs before, during, and after any exercise session. By adding a glucose load after your workout, as many believe is essential, you lose some of the insulin-sensitizing benefits of the exercise.[11] In a study published in 2022,[12] scientists recruited seven women to do a workout, after which one group ate nothing and the other ate carbs (or actually drank them—a typical energy drink). The researchers also monitored the glucose control of the women the following day by feeding them identical diets. In the women who exercised and ate nothing afterward, their glucose levels throughout the next day were low and stable. In the women who exercised and then had the energy drink, glucose levels were much more variable and higher than expected.

Protein, Fat, Carbs—and Calories

As we said earlier, the food you eat can be the culprit or the cure. There are numerous other variables that contribute to insulin resistance, such as lack of exercise, stress, and poor sleep; we'll explore those in the coming chapters. However, even if you're managing each of these well, but you continue to eat in a manner that keeps your insulin elevated, you won't have the success you want. In contrast, managing insulin through smart eating will absolutely make up for other variables not being buttoned down. For example, if you're eating well, the fact that you can't exercise as often as you should matters much, much less.

The insulin-sensitizing plans that follow work by targeting insulin resistance at its likely starting point: in your fat cells. (Part of this discussion will touch on excess body weight and obesity, but we don't necessarily want to frame it in that context because—as you'll know if you read *Why We Get Sick*—body weight is just one aspect of overall health that is affected by insulin resistance. Preventing chronic disease is paramount. So let's let weight be tangential. That said, if your goal for reading this book is to lose or control your weight, there is of course lots for you here too.) Shrinking a fat cell is built on two fundamental ideas: low insulin and low energy (which is to say, low calories).

Hydrate, Hydrate!

While we don't recommend reaching for an energy drink after you work out (or any other time!), we can't stress enough how important it is to hydrate. One of the most consistent findings across populations is that underhydration (not quite dehydration, but close) is a foundational feature of poor metabolic health. In fact, people who are chronically underhydrated are over four times more likely to die compared with those who are adequately hydrated, and this includes deaths from diseases derivative of insulin resistance.[1] In fact, insulin resistance is among the strongest predictors of being underhydrated—in other words, if you have insulin resistance, you are likely underhydrated.

When our bodies are underhydrated, our blood is too concentrated with minerals, such as sodium and others. There's tremendous benefit to getting adequate minerals in our diet. However, if the minerals outpace the water in our blood, forcing the blood to become too concentrated with minerals, we begin creating metabolic problems.

On average, people with insulin resistance have concentrated blood. (Interestingly, by simply increasing blood mineral concentration with intravenous infusions, researchers can force insulin resistance in people,[2] even down to the level of individual cells.) So do drink lots of insulin-friendly fluids: of course water, but also unsweetened tea, sparkling water (a personal favorite), and even diet soda. How much water you need to ensure proper hydration is very individualized. Depending on climate and exercise habits, it's impossible to have a single rule. In general, you should be drinking enough water that your urine is clear at least one time that day. And don't wait until you feel thirsty!

Low Insulin Shrinks Fat Cells

Insulin controls the size of a fat cell, but how it does so is often misunderstood. It doesn't promote growth per se—that is, it doesn't push more fat into the fat cell—but rather it inhibits fat breakdown.

Let's use the analogy of a sink. Insulin isn't opening the tap and increasing the water coming into the sink from the faucet, but rather, it's closing up the drain, leading the sink to fill up. When insulin is low, the fat cell shrinks because the drain is open wide; water can drain out faster than new water is coming in.

While insulin doesn't open the "faucet" any wider, it *is* absolutely essential in telling the fat cell what to do with the energy coming in. Whether it's fats or glucose coming in from the blood, insulin tells the fat cell what to do with it— namely, store it as triglycerides. (Yes, fat cells are perfectly capable of turning glucose into stored fat . . . but only if insulin is elevated.) If insulin stays high, it wants to hoard energy in the fat cells, which means there's less energy available in the blood (likely a reason why insulin promotes hunger: the body senses less energy is available and wants to take in more).

When insulin is low, however, the body is so eager to *use* energy that it mobilizes numerous metabolic processes in an effort to burn what it's been storing:

- When insulin stays low after a meal, available energy in the blood is higher and, not surprisingly, hunger is abated.[13]
- With low insulin, the body actually increases its metabolic rate by roughly 300 calories per day![14] This could manifest in both a slightly higher body temperature and more spontaneous movement, like fidgeting.
- When insulin is low, certain cells of the body, burning fat at a very high rate, produce ketones, and these ketones are wasted from the body in the breath and urine.

Altogether, these variables are why a low-insulin state facilitates the shrinking of fat cells.

Low Energy Shrinks Fat Cells

There is no doubt that calories matter when it comes to shrinking fat cells. That said, you really can't separate a reduction in energy from a reduction in insulin. (If you cut calories but somehow managed to keep insulin elevated, you would quickly become unconscious. Insulin wants to store energy, but if insufficient calories are coming, it has nothing to store and, thus, drops. If insulin were high without sufficient energy, the amount of available nutrients in the blood would drop to a potentially dangerous level—hence the loss of consciousness!) By reducing energy coming in, the body is forced to increasingly rely on its own stored energy.

Fat cells are the greatest energy storage in the body, and it's not even close. The body has about 2,000 calories stored as glycogen (the storage form of glucose) but, even in a lean individual, it has well over 100 times that amount stored as energy. So, long after the liver has used up all its glycogen, the fat cells continually provide their energy to the body, breaking down triglycerides into free fatty acids to be burned directly for energy or converted into ketones.

What About Alcohol?

We've said that there are three macronutrients: fat, protein, and carbs. Actually, there is a fourth: alcohol.

While it's (obviously!) not an essential nutrient, alcohol does have calories, which is a main parameter for something being considered a macro. Beyond delivering extra calories, however, alcohol intake should be limited or avoided if your goal is to prevent or reverse insulin resistance or maintain insulin sensitivity.

When alcohol enters the body, it insists on being burned first.[1] This is partly because, unlike dietary fats and carbohydrates, alcohol cannot be stored in the body. When it comes in, it gets metabolized for energy.

However, only the liver can metabolize alcohol. The rest of the body can't help because only the liver has the necessary enzymes.[2] The liver gets overwhelmed by this metabolic burden and is often unable to do the job completely. When this happens, instead of burning the alcohol for energy, the liver turns that excess alcohol into fat.[3] That fat steadily accumulates in the liver, eventually turning into fatty liver disease.[4]

Meanwhile, because alcohol has taken metabolic priority, whatever other nutrients are either already in the blood (high blood glucose), or that come with the alcohol (such as sugar), have to wait to be burned. If they end up with nowhere to go, they eventually will be stored as fats where they are rather than being burned for energy. This leads to fat accumulating in tissues that are ill suited to long-term fat storage, such as the liver and muscles,[5] which, as we have seen, leads to insulin resistance.

The obvious solution is to limit your alcohol intake. If you do decide to imbibe, consider the sugar/carbohydrate content of your drink. Most beer, wine, cider, and mixed drinks have carbs (straight liquor does not, but it does still have calories). For tracking your macros, alcohol can be lumped in with your carb intake simply because alcohol so often comes with sugar of some kind—either sugar directly or some juice.

Reverse
Percent of Calories

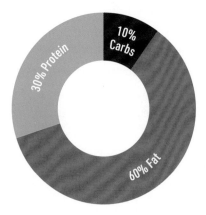

Prevent
Percent of Calories

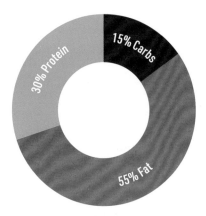

Maintain
Percent of Calories

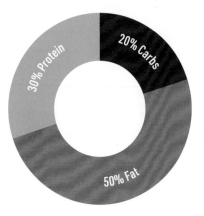

How We'll Put It into Action

With all of this in mind, let's review the general dietary suggestions relevant to each of the three strategies: Reverse, Prevent, and Maintain. You'll notice a pattern—while protein remains stable, the balance of carbohydrates to fat is shifting:

❋ Reverse: 60% fat, 30% protein, 10% carb
❋ Prevent: 55% fat, 30% protein, 15% carb
❋ Maintain: 50% fat, 30% protein, 20% carb

One note: These caloric breakdowns aren't meant to be absolute. As important as it is to control dietary carbohydrates, the amount *can* be increased slightly if you exercise a lot.

To track your macros, we recommend that you download an app, which will make this math much easier (in that the app will actually do the macro math for you). Our favorite is Avatar Nutrition.

The Power of Movement

This is probably the least controversial point we'll make: exercising is a good way to improve your metabolic health. From children to the elderly, in both males and females, exercise improves insulin resistance.[1] But it might be a challenge to put that knowledge into practice.

Diana has been coaching clients long enough to know that there's an imaginary divide in many people's minds: the "fitness people" and the "regular people." So many times, a new client will say that they "just aren't one of those fitness people" and seem to force themselves through every workout.

We've got to break it to you: you *are* one of those fitness people. You are living in a human body that is composed of muscles and a heart and a pair of lungs. You've heard the phrase "use it or lose it," and that applies here: unless you can find a way to opt out of having a physical body, then you've got to work what you have in order to make it stronger, more functional, and a more comfortable place to reside—and to improve insulin sensitivity. You don't have to do uncomfortable workouts or to oil yourself up and get onstage or take bikini photos, but you should update your concept of yourself as someone who exercises regularly. That's you now!

So, Someone Who Exercises Regularly, this chapter is all about understanding the underlying power of exercise and what really happens when you move your body. It might just be the motivation you need to get going.

You Can Start Small

Before we go any further, we want to drive home one point. When it comes to exercise, a little goes a long way. For example, even walking every day for a few weeks is enough to improve insulin sensitivity in people with insulin resistance.[2] In fact, just moving is so helpful that the body becomes more insulin sensitive even in the absence of any weight changes.[3] So while we will recommend training your muscles, really, the most important thing is that you *just move*. You can work your way up to greater challenges.

Muscle Matters

At the risk of seeming silly by defining it, exercise is a period of time wherein the muscles engage in repetitive and exhausting movement. We're saying that to emphasize the role of skeletal muscle. When it comes to managing metabolic health, muscle is the undeniable winner.

While insulin resistance likely starts in fat cells, it can be subtle (and clinically undetected with conventional tests) until it reaches the muscle. At that point, things get more dramatic and obvious. Keeping muscles insulin sensitive is not only a good way to prevent the problem from going too far but also a way to reverse course and take the fight back to the fat cells.

Muscle constitutes almost half of the tissue mass of the average individual (though some people do have more fat mass than muscle). When the muscles begin moving, the muscle cells' metabolic rate increases dramatically. Increased metabolic rate really just means increased fuel demand. This increased demand is helpful in a general sense for improving insulin resistance: overfat fat cells that can share their fat with working muscle cells are able to shrink, thus addressing a root cause of insulin resistance. In addition, the working muscle has a high demand for glucose (and every other fuel source). Naturally, this helps control insulin.

In fact, the working muscle is so determined to get enough fuel to maintain its efforts that it gets that fuel (glucose) through a "back door." Normally, at rest, a muscle gets glucose only if insulin allows it. When glucose rises after a meal, insulin will climb in response to help turn the glucose curve back down to normal. To do this, insulin will bind to muscle cells and elicit a series of events, one of which is to open glucose transporters. Once open, the glucose transporters allow the glucose to come rushing into the muscle cells, thereby lowering blood glucose and providing energy to the muscle. When energy demand is elevated, as is the case during exercise, the working muscle can't rely on insulin, and the muscle cell opens the glucose transporters without insulin's help—in other words, exercise provides an insulin-independent mechanism for fueling the muscle with glucose. In a nutshell, this is why moving your muscles matters so much.

The insulin-independent pathway is essential to the muscle because insulin is antithetical to exercise. Remember, insulin is the hormone of the "fed state" and accordingly wants to store energy. During exercise, the body isn't interested in *storing* energy, but rather *using* it, mobilizing stored energy from liver and fat cells in order to give it to the working muscle cells. All of this means insulin is forced to take a back seat. A fascinating reason for this is that insulin wants to feed *all* cells, but why would we want fat cells to be fed when we want them to share their "food" with other cells? Indeed, it would create such a competition for energy across all cells that the working muscle cells that are pulling the load (perhaps literally) would lack the needed energy to maintain the effort for any real period of time. In

Does Muscle Have a Sweet Tooth?

Working muscle uses a lot of glucose, but that isn't necessarily a matter of preference, as we often think. People are quick to state that the working muscle "prefers glucose," but this isn't quite accurate. The muscle cell will use what's available—glucose, yes, but also fat or ketones. At lower intensities of exercise, muscles use fat as the primary fuel, but as intensity increases, the muscles switch to glucose. This is more a matter of oxygen availability than any true "preference." Unlike glucose, fats and ketones must be metabolized ("burned") in the mitochondria through a process that requires a high degree of oxygen (known as oxidative metabolism). During exercise, especially as intensity goes up, the muscle has a hard time getting enough oxygen—blood flow just can't keep up with the muscle's demands. Not only does this lead to the accumulation of things like lactate and hydrogen (the latter affecting the pH of the muscle and causing the "burning" sensation) but it also means there's insufficient oxygen to light the fat- and ketone-burning flame. Glucose is also metabolized in the mitochondria, but unlike the other fuels, it can act as a hybrid fuel, metabolized *outside* the mitochondria (a process known as nonoxidative glycolysis, for all you scientists out there). The ability to be used without oxygen gives glucose a competitive advantage and allows the muscle to continue its work in the lower-oxygen environment that intense exercise creates.

other words, while insulin wants to feed both fat cells and muscle cells, during exercise, we want the fat cells to help feed the muscle cells.

Exercise and Other Hormones

The need to *use*, not *store*, energy is so urgent that there are several hormones that spring into action during exercise to ensure that happens. Perhaps the most powerful is epinephrine (a.k.a. adrenaline). Epinephrine is involved in essentially every process related to exercise, including increasing heart rate and blood pressure (to make sure blood is moving quickly and feeding the muscles), inducing sweat (to help maintain body temperature), and, most relevant to this discussion, increasing fuel availability. Epinephrine has direct effects on fat cells (by stimulating lipolysis) and liver cells (by stimulating lipolysis and glycogenolysis), increasing their fuel-sharing tendencies.

To help it mobilize energy, epinephrine knows that insulin needs to be stopped. So it takes the fight for energy directly to the beta cells of the pancreas, the site of insulin production. When epinephrine comes to the beta cells, it initiates a series of events within the cell that not only inhibits insulin production but also inhibits its release—doing everything it can to ensure that insulin doesn't come along and ruin its plan to keep the muscle fueled.

In addition to producing insulin-sensitizing hormones, exercise also helps address the canonical causes of insulin resistance. As noted, it helps lower insulin, but it also lowers stress and inflammation, the *primary* drivers of insulin resistance. That exercise improves all three should be all the motivation you need to get started.

Beyond epinephrine, other hormones help create an insulin-sensitizing environment during exercise. Like so many tissues these days, the muscle is now recognized as an endocrine organ. We used to have a short list of endocrine organs, such as the thyroid gland, adrenal glands, or gonads. However, we now know that almost every tissue (likely every tissue indeed) actively produces and secretes hormones into the blood. Muscle is no exception and is in fact a heavy producer of multiple hormones—the group referred to as the myokines. Two in particular are worthy of mention here: irisin and FGF21.

Irisin and FGF21 are both produced by working muscles. In addition to sharing a common origin, they share some helpful metabolic effects at the fat cells. Each of these myokines is capable of making low-metabolic storage-mode fat cells behave like higher-metabolic burn-mode fat cells. Not only do they stimulate greater mitochondrial biogenesis in the fat cells (which increases glucose and fat burning) but they also shrink the size of the fat droplets in the fat cells, effectively shrinking the fat cell. Collectively, these actions serve to increase fat-cell insulin sensitivity. To varying degrees, irisin and FGF21 go further by enhancing insulin sensitivity in the liver and even the muscle itself (this latter effect is known as "autocrine" signaling—when a hormone produced by a cell signals back to the very cell that made it).

Use It or Lose It

If all of this isn't sufficient motivation, here's more to help light the fire. By not working your muscles, you're not only losing out on the insulin-sensitizing benefit of exercise, but you're actually making insulin resistance *worse*. Think about your activity before eating. Are you sitting around a lot or moving about? If you've been sitting still before eating, as opposed to occasionally interrupting the sitting, the blood glucose response to your meal will be about double what it would otherwise be.[4] Furthermore, being sedentary for a few days causes demonstrable insulin resistance even in otherwise healthy people,[5] and the problem only gets worse with age.[6] An effective and simple solution to prevent insulin resistance with inactivity is to simply flex the muscles from time to time; contracting a muscle 30 times for just a few seconds at a time is enough to help lower the risk of insulin resistance.[7]

But just flexing some muscles while sitting won't get you all the benefits that regular (challenging) exercise has to offer, so for those who are ready to do more, let's get into specifics.

What Kind of Exercise?

There are many types of exercise, but for simplicity's sake we'll consider two broad categories: aerobic and resistance. First is aerobic exercise, also known as a "cardio workout," where you are moving briskly to get your heart rate pumping. The second is resistance exercise, where you are working specific muscles to strengthen them. The majority of research conducted on the topic of exercise and insulin resistance has focused on aerobic exercise, though resistance exercise has also been studied enough for us to make the firm conclusion that it also helps. Again, none of this is surprising—moving the body improves insulin resistance.

If we compare aerobic and resistance exercise head-to-head, resistance training may be superior in improving insulin sensitivity at the lower end of a time range (say, 1 hour per week), though as duration increases (2+ hours per week), the differences wash out.[8] So, if you're pressed for time, resistance exercise will yield better results in less time—which is why we focus on it in chapter 12.

That resistance exercise may improve insulin sensitivity more than aerobic exercise (such as running) is largely a function of the changes in muscle mass across the two types of exercise;[9] resistance training increases muscle mass, while aerobic generally does not.[10] More muscle means more glucose consumption and more favorable myokines.

One common reason people prefer aerobic exercise over resistance exercise may be the simplicity of it. For effective aerobic exercise, you simply need to get up and get going. Whether it's a brisk walk or a bike ride, your goal is to increase your heart rate. Resistance training is a bit more complicated, involving sets, reps, grips, angles, and motions that may be unfamiliar. (Don't worry: the plan that we outline later in the book will help with all of this!)

A fundamental principle with effective resistance training is to work the muscles in their respective complementary groups. You can essentially separate all exercises into two key motions: pushing and pulling. This admittedly simple scheme allows training to follow natural, functional movement and promotes complementary muscle development. For example, many people love to do biceps curls, which strengthen the biceps alone. But strong biceps are largely useless if your back muscles are weak; every real-world motion that involves the biceps (any motion in which the elbow closes) involves back muscles as well. Similarly, rather than focusing on an exercise that challenges only the triceps (the back of the arm), you "push" (either a weight or your own body), which allows the triceps to be worked with the chest, its natural partner in movement.

These kinds of exercises do not require a gym membership. You can perform all kinds of combinations of exercises with just your body weight. Where that's an awkward challenge, you can include the use of even modest weights or other devices (like water jugs).

An unfortunate tendency with resistance exercise is to focus on the upper body and overlook the lower body. Perhaps the fact that our legs are often hidden under our pants makes it easy to ignore them (not that we're suggesting you stop wearing pants), while our arms are often on display. However, don't let this distract you. You will have *much* better success controlling and maintaining insulin sensitivity by ensuring your legs get exercised (and exhausted), more so than your arms. Simply put—don't waste time with exercises that only work your arms. Spend that time on working your legs. Though your sore legs may mean you walk a little funny the next day, the improvements in your insulin sensitivity will be no joke.

Bottom line: Don't think that resistance training is not for you. Remember that 1 hour of resistance exercise in a week can improve insulin resistance more than 1 hour of aerobic exercise.[11]

In the Zone

Regarding aerobic exercise specifically, a great deal of attention recently has focused on training zones. Training zones aren't a new concept, but they're getting much more attention in recent years due to social media. In particular, many advocate training in "zone 2," which is a moderately challenging state—essentially that sweet spot where you're exercising but can still carry on a conversation. There's no doubt zone 2 is an interesting spot, as it stands at a metabolic balance point between glucose and fat reliance. At lower intensities, muscles use fat as the primary fuel, but as intensity increases, the muscles switch to glucose (see "Do Muscles Have a Sweet Tooth?" on page 63). Essentially, zone 2 is the spot at which the muscles are *just* about to switch to glucose, pressing the muscle's ability to rely on fat as far as it can go, but not further. Because of this, many espouse the idea that zone 2 is the best for inducing the creation of new mitochondria ("mitochondrial biogenesis"), and some have claimed that zone 2 is best for improving insulin resistance. Both of these claims *may* be true, but there is little published evidence to support it. Nevertheless, as stated above, any exercise is better than none!

How Intense Should My Workout Be?

The harder you can exercise, the greater the improvement in insulin sensitivity.[12] Of course, don't go harder than you can. But if you are able to work harder during your exercise, it pays dividends even greater than the length of time you exercise.[13] Increasing the intensity, despite a shorter time (~20 minutes), is at least as effective at correcting insulin resistance as lower-intensity, longer-duration exercise.[14]

When implementing high-intensity training, start out with less intense challenges and gradually work up to higher intensities. For aerobic exercise, high-intensity workouts are achieved by simply performing the exercise more

Post-exercise cool down/ warm up

Often, when available, people enjoy a sauna or even an ice bath after exercise. Whether this is part of your routine or not, it's worth briefly highlighting the metabolic impact of "thermal stress."

With heat, when internal body temperature starts to climb, even by less than 1°C, blood vessels widen dramatically (known as "vasodilation") in an effort to cool down. But at the same time, more blood begins to flow through muscle tissue, leading to greater muscle glucose uptake, which helps lower glucose and keeps insulin better in check.[1]

On the opposite end of the thermostat, cold therapy has been shown to have similar insulin-sensitizing benefits, albeit through completely different mechanisms. When the body gets cold, the main cellular response is to shiver. As with exercise, when the muscle is working, even shivering, it has insulin-independent means to pull glucose in from the blood, thereby lowering blood glucose and insulin. At the same, the body is so determined to stay warm that it recruits fat cells to help. Fat cells have the remarkable ability to become little heaters, burning glucose to make heat. Altogether, the shivering muscles and the "warm" fat cells help lower blood glucose, which in turn brings insulin down, thereby improving insulin sensitivity.

vigorously. An ideal way to do this is interval training, where a period of lower-intensity exercise is followed by a period of higher intensity, then repeated for the desired duration. For resistance exercise, higher intensity is achieved by repeating a series of motions until you can't do any more. This approach is surprisingly effective—just a few exercises performed one single time to exhaustion carries substantial insulin-sensitizing effects.[15]

When Should I Work Out?

There are two answers to this question. The first: not only are we actually stronger and faster in the afternoon, but an afternoon workout has distinct metabolic benefits as well. A 12-week training study had subjects with insulin resistance go through exercise sessions either in the morning (sometime between 8 and 10 a.m.) or afternoon (sometime between 3 and 6 p.m.). The afternoon session resulted in significant improvements in multiple indicators of insulin resistance, and, as noted, they performed better.[16] It's unclear exactly why that time frame was superior, but it is likely a consequence of being able to simply exercise "better"—because the body is more warmed up in the afternoon, we are able to work out with more intensity, and intensity matters when it comes to improving insulin resistance.

That brings us to the second answer, though. Even though there may be slightly lower metabolic benefit to exercising in the morning, it's also often better for consistency—there are usually relatively fewer distractions in the morning than the afternoon. But maybe the only time you can fit in a workout is in the evening after your children have gone to bed. So really, the best time to exercise is whenever you can.

Stress and Sleep

There are many variables that contribute to insulin resistance—too many to explain, and without much need because many of them have such a modest influence. We consider a cause of insulin resistance to be "primary" if it meets two criteria:

1. It can cause insulin resistance on its own, without any other stimulus.
2. It has been shown to cause insulin resistance in all three commonly used biomedical models (isolated cell cultures, laboratory rodents, and humans).

This is a strict definition, but it helps cut through what might otherwise be distraction. After we've used this filter, we're left with three primary causes. In the previous chapters, we've already explored two: chronically elevated insulin and inflammation. But we haven't talked yet about the third: stress.

The Metabolic Consequences of Stress

To understand the role of stress in insulin resistance, we need to have a common understanding of what stress is. Simply put, stress that impacts insulin resistance is a problem of the two prototypical stress hormones—cortisol and epinephrine (a.k.a. adrenaline). Ensuring that these two hormones stay in their proper place is a key part of preventing insulin resistance.

Cortisol and epinephrine have little in common. They're made in different cells, have very different molecular structures, and act at different parts of the body. However, they do share one very important attribute—they both seek to increase blood glucose levels.

Cortisol is particularly determined to see the body flush with glucose, and will signal to the liver to make glucose out of almost anything, including lactate (the primary building block), glycerol (from breaking down stored fat), and amino acids (from protein). Its goal is to ensure that the body has enough glucose to fuel metabolic processes to get through what you perceive to be a stressful situation, whether that's running away from a predator, having relationship troubles, or staying up late studying.

Epinephrine is the first responder to a stressful situation and is responsible for the obvious cardiovascular effects we notice, like increased heart rate and sweaty palms. However, like cortisol, epinephrine will elicit a rise in blood glucose, and while it's also acting on the liver, it's sending a different signal. Whereas cortisol pushes the liver to make new glucose from any circulating building blocks, epinephrine primarily signals the liver to simply release the glucose that it has stored, breaking down glycogen.

Naturally, these glucose-pushing hormones are at odds with insulin, which is now working harder than ever to keep that glucose under control. And this is where the metabolic mayhem occurs (one of the very rare instances in which insulin loses ground). The stress response was such an important survival mechanism (at least, in the days when it was more common for us humans to encounter life-or-death situations, like running from a bear) that insulin can't compete. Collectively, the stress hormones win the nutrient battle for glucose and the body becomes insulin resistant as long as those hormones are elevated.

How to Keep Stress Hormones Under Control

Obviously, there are many contributors to stress in our lives. There are also many resources that aim to help individuals cope with stress—and what works for one person might not help another. (For instance, some of you might swear by yoga, while others turn to a relaxing stroll; someone else might benefit from a long soak in the tub, while someone else might call a friend.) So we'll keep this chapter pretty short and focus on two strategies that would work for just about everyone.

The most important and valuable habit to lower cortisol and epinephrine is to improve your sleep habits. Everybody knows that sleep is important for numerous aspects of good health, but few appreciate its potent effects on insulin resistance.

When we sleep poorly, we experience a significant and meaningful increase in stress hormones the next day—after all, sleep deprivation is a stressor. This change carries a rapidly noticeable metabolic effect. Just one week of poor sleep will increase insulin resistance by about 30%.[1] Even more sobering is the fact that just two days of sleep restriction can cause demonstrable insulin resistance.[2]

But—as too many of us know—getting more, better sleep is easier said than done. So to help, here are two points of attack to make that goal a reality.

The first is well known: reducing light exposure in the evening. Blue light is the aspect of light that has the greatest effect on these matters. You may have heard of blue light. It is notoriously the type of light that our TVs, laptops, and smartphones emit. Fluorescent and LED lights also give off blue light—and so does the sun. That's why blue light can be either friend or foe. When we're exposed to blue light in the evening, our levels of the sleep hormone melatonin will be altered, potentially compromising sleep. The light itself is a stress in the evening, increasing cortisol levels throughout the night.[3] Blue light exposure during the day, however, can actually *mitigate* the cortisol-spiking effect of poor sleep![4] In general, then, you want to harness the power of blue light wisely, deliberately exposing yourself to it during the day, and reducing it in the evening. In other words, try to mimic the pattern of light exposure you'd get from the sun. This means limiting your exposure to those blue light–emitting screens in the evening; ideally,

> Just one week of poor sleep will increase insulin resistance by about 30%. Just two days of sleep restriction can cause demonstrable insulin resistance.

no screens within about two hours of going to bed. If it seems like too much of a challenge to quit cold turkey, try to baby-step your way into it by skipping your evening TV or social media check-ins a couple of nights a week and work your way up. (As an added bonus, avoiding the news cycle and stopping the late-night doomscrolling may also decrease your stress level, beyond improving sleep!)

The second strategy to improve sleep is less known, but much more potent: not spiking blood glucose before bed. Increased blood glucose causes increased body heat, and elevated body temperature is a common cause of insomnia. This is likely why eating a high-carbohydrate meal or snack before bed leads to such poor sleep.[5]

(Of course, our culture of sitting in front of the TV and eating treats every evening creates a perfect storm.) This is accomplished by following the eating strategies outlined in chapters 2, 3, 4, and 5: either fasting after your evening meal or (if you must have a snack later) making it one that won't spike glucose. Chapter 13 has some options for you.

A final component of a plan to prevent insulin resistance is to manage stress through proper breathing. A common practice is diaphragmatic breathing, or "belly" breathing. Setting aside time for mindful periods of belly breathing has a significant dampening effect on stress hormones.[6] Our suggestion is to practice this breathing for 10 minutes daily, ideally without any stimulation—that is, no TV, no book, nothing but you and your breath.

A Simple Belly Breathing Exercise

Find a comfortable position, such as sitting in a supportive chair or lying in bed. Make sure your head and neck are relaxed and comfortable. Place one hand on your belly, just below your rib cage, and the other on your chest. With your lips closed, slowly inhale through your nose and try to send your breath deep into your belly. You should feel the hand on your belly rise as your diaphragm expands, while the hand on your chest should move very little. Tighten your abdominal muscles as you slowly exhale through your mouth and feel the hand on your belly fall. Repeat.

The Plan

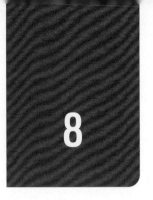

8

Reverse

Most people reading this book will want to start their new insulin sensitizing lifestyle here, with the plan to Reverse. We're confident in that claim because the overwhelming majority of adults are insulin resistant.

You're ready to begin the fight against insulin resistance through that two-pronged strategy we outlined in the first part of this book. That said, we don't recommend that you jump into restricting calories right away (or at least don't make it your primary focus). Simply put, starting by cutting calories leads to hunger. If your insulin-sensitizing journey is based on cutting energy, you might be tempted to eat less and exercise more. While this can work in the (very) short term, you will unwittingly be pitting yourself against hunger, and in our environment of readily accessible food, hunger always wins. So we'll start by lowering insulin.

Lowering insulin and (eventually) energy is best achieved with two complementary strategies—a low-carbohydrate diet and intermittent fasting.

On the Reverse track, you'll aim to get 60 percent of your daily caloric intake from fat, 30 percent from protein, and 10 percent from carbohydrates. In addition, aim for less than 50 grams of net carbohydrates per day (at least at first). This will very likely have a ketogenic effect. Remember that ketones are simply pieces of fat burning, which is a positive sign that insulin is low. Indeed, it might be helpful to monitor your success by measuring your ketones daily (see Testing at Home, page 20). If you detect ketones in your breath, urine, or blood, you can be very confident your insulin levels are in a good range.

While controlling carbohydrates is vital to reversing insulin resistance, if you're exercising a lot—if you're diligent about running or lifting weights for 30 to 60 minutes a day—you will absolutely be able to eat more than 50 grams of net carbohydrates in a day and remain in ketosis. Unfortunately, it's hard to know how much more you can eat, but suffice it to say that the 50-gram limit can be more loosely adhered to. Monitoring your ketones will help you determine the right amount for you.

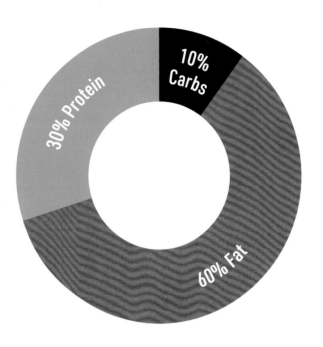

Reverse
Percent of Calories

10% Carbs

30% Protein

60% Fat

For truly rapid results, control carbohydrates by focusing on low-glycemic-load foods and limiting the amount of carbohydrate foods you eat (as outlined in chapter 5). Focus on low-sugar fruits and especially vegetables. Don't forget: eat them, don't drink them—no juices or smoothies.

When you start on a low-carb diet, you should not be focused on restricting energy—don't go hungry. *After* you've learned to lower insulin through the principles outlined in chapters 3, 4, and 5, *then* you can turn your attention to lowering energy consumption. (As mentioned earlier, when insulin is lower, hunger is, too, which makes restricting calories less of a challenge.)

However, you don't have to push the plate away at mealtime while you're still hungry in an effort to cut back on the amount of energy you're consuming. Instead, you can use intermittent fasting (which, as you now know, helps keep insulin low, in addition to cutting out some calories). Avoid the temptation to count calories or monitor the amount of energy you burn during exercise. Simply avoid energy during a fasting window and eat normally (until satiated) when it's time. Revisit chapter 2 to choose a strategy for incorporating fasting into your daily or weekly routine. The meal plan that follows offers breakfast suggestions for every day of the week, and you can add fasting over breakfast when you feel ready.

Exercise or engage in some kind of vigorous activity most days of the week. Whether this is a challenging walk (on the border of having to break into a run) or lifting weights (or your own body), make sure you're working hard. This is particularly important if you hope to gain and maintain muscle.

Remember, even if you're older, you can still significantly increase the size of your muscles by working them to exhaustion. Of course, the older we are, the more careful we want to be in pushing a joint too hard for fear of injury. Thankfully, the evidence suggests that even when doing more repetitions with a lighter weight, if the activity is performed to the point that the muscle is exhausted (that is, you can't do any more), you will have the same increase in muscle as if you used a heavier weight and performed fewer repetitions.

When to Move On

Eventually, you'll be ready for your metabolic graduation from Reverse to Prevent. Of course, an obvious method to gauge your current status is to repeat the blood tests mentioned in chapter 1, or use the DIY methods as a tracker. Alternatively, here are three items to look for as signs of progress:

1. Weight loss around the abdomen: Central fat storage contributes more toward insulin resistance, and as you narrow your waist, that's strong evidence that you're reversing insulin resistance.

2. Skin improvements: Not everyone manifests insulin resistance with skin tags, but they're a great indicator to keep an eye on. If you're turning back the metabolic clock, these should be improving, if they haven't left entirely.

3. Blood pressure: Insulin has a strong influence on salt and water balance in the body, and when insulin is high, blood pressure most certainly will be as well. If your blood pressure has improved to a normal range, it's a very strong indicator that you're ready to make a lifestyle change that reflects your improved metabolic state.

A Note on Blood Pressure

If you've had insulin resistance for some time (and likely long before you knew you had it), you almost certainly have high blood pressure. We won't explore here the multiple ways in which insulin resistance forces a higher blood pressure (if you're interested, see *Why We Get Sick*), but one of the central mechanisms is the effect of insulin on how the body handles sodium. Normally, the body keeps blood sodium in a very narrow range, and it does this by regulating the amount of water in the blood. When insulin is low, the kidneys are free to regulate this in an optimal manner, letting excess sodium be excreted in the urine, and taking any excess water with it. As the water leaves the blood, it helps maintain a normal blood pressure. However, when insulin is elevated, it forces the kidneys (via other hormones) to retain sodium, which then forces the retention of water. Now there's too much water in the blood, and when blood volume increases, so too does pressure.

As insulin resistance is reversed and insulin levels come down (and they will), the kidneys are able to finally remove all the extra sodium and water that have been in the blood. As this happens, blood pressure can begin to drop quickly—in fact, so quickly that if you're taking blood pressure medications, your blood pressure may be dangerously low. So be sure to keep in contact with your clinical team throughout this metabolic transition in case changes in blood pressure medications are needed. And of course, be sure to drink plenty of water and don't shy away from salt (remember: too little salt can actually cause insulin resistance!). These habits will help prevent blood pressure from dropping too much too quickly.

REVERSE MEAL PLAN (10% CARBS)

	Breakfast	Lunch	Dinner
MONDAY	Classic Omelet, page 139 (or fasting)	Creamy Dill Tuna Salad, page 152	Easy Chicken Enchilada Casserole, page 165
TUESDAY	Cheesy Sausage and Egg Casserole, page 132 (or fasting)	leftover Easy Chicken Enchilada Casserole, page 165	Fully Loaded Cheeseburger Skillet, page 186
WEDNESDAY	Baked Puffy Pancake, page 131 (or fasting)	leftover Fully Loaded Cheeseburger Skillet, page 186	Mediterranean Turkey Bowls, page 171
THURSDAY	Your New Favorite Breakfast Burrito, page 136 (or fasting)	leftover Mediterranean Turkey Bowls, page 171	Meatzza Pizza, page 153
FRIDAY	Fluffy Pancakes, page 128 (or fasting)	Ground Beef Taco Salad, page 150	Creamy Garlic Shrimp, page 194, and The Best Broccoli, page 216
SATURDAY	hard-boiled eggs and raw almonds (or fasting)	leftover Creamy Garlic Shrimp, page 194, and The Best Broccoli, page 216	Favorite Lamb Larb, page 172, and Better-Than-Mashed-Potatoes, page 214
SUNDAY	Egg-Cheddar-Ham Sandwich, page 135 (or fasting)	Caesar Salad with Seasoned Chicken, page 149	Grilled Sunday Steak, page 185, and Stir-Fried Rice, page 213

Notes: Begin and end each day with 2 tablespoons apple cider vinegar upon waking and before bed.

These meal plans are meant to be used simply as a suggestion, and portion sizes should be determined based on your overall caloric needs. While each dish may not fit the target carb count, the meal will hit the target when considering all of the dishes in combination. For example, Sunday's dinner of steak and stir-fried rice hits the target of 10% since the steak contains 0% carbs while the rice contains 20% carbs, which balances out to 10% carbs.

9

Prevent

The Prevent track is intended for people who are at a sort of metabolic tipping point. As mentioned in earlier chapters, you might be here because you are currently only mildly insulin resistant—on the precipice of sliding down the hill into the bog of deep insulin resistance. Others of you have endured the struggle of climbing the slope and coming out of insulin resistance—though you might easily slip back into it. Regardless of how you got to the tipping point, this plan is intended to get you back onto the stable ground of insulin sensitivity and further from the edge.

The Reverse track strategy to keep fat cells in check via low insulin and low energy (see the previous chapter) still generally applies in the Prevent track—this is essential in climbing the metabolic hill in the first place—though your targets will shift.

On this plan you have a higher allowance for dietary carbohydrate than if you're seeking to reverse insulin resistance, but not much. Stick to a range of around 15% of calories from carbohydrates, 55% from fat, and 30% from protein. Ideally, those carbs should come from low-starch vegetables and low-sugar fruit, which will help ensure that insulin isn't spiked too often.

Revisit chapter 2 to find a strategy for intermittent fasting that you can

Prevent
Percent of Calories

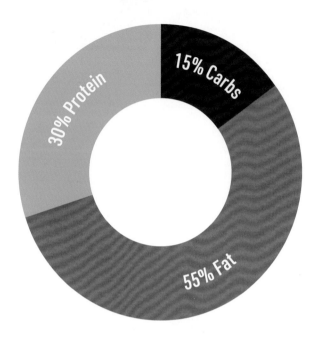

15% Carbs

55% Fat

30% Protein

incorporate into your daily or weekly routine. Or use the model in the sample weekly meal plan that follows, which builds in morning fasts three times a week.

Exercise or engage in some kind of vigorous activity most days of the week. Whether this is a challenging walk (on the border of having to break into a run) or lifting weights (or your own body), make sure you're working hard. This is particularly important if you hope to gain and maintain muscle.

Remember, even if you're older, you can still significantly increase the size of your muscles by working them to exhaustion. Of course, the older we are, the more careful we want to be in pushing a joint too hard for fear of injury. Thankfully, the evidence suggests that even when doing more repetitions with a lighter weight, if the activity is performed to the point that the muscle is exhausted (that is, you can't do any more), you will have the same increase in muscle as if you used a heavier weight and performed fewer repetitions.

The Prevent phase is an interesting one. For many, this a phase where you simply pass through (i.e., improving insulin resistance). However, for others, this phase lasts a lifetime; thanks to genetics (such as how you store fat in fat cells), some people will have an ongoing struggle with insulin resistance. Because this is a more subtle stage, relying on the same markers outlined in the "graduation" from Reverse to Prevent might not work. In this case, you can rely on ketones as a marker. We're *not* suggesting you need to adopt a ketogenic diet, but ketones are markers of insulin levels, albeit inversely (that is, when insulin is low, ketones start to climb). So conduct an experiment: eat dinner around 6 p.m., following our general dietary guidelines. Fast through breakfast the next day, and then around noon, measure your ketones with a ketone meter. If your ketone levels are around 0.3 mM, that's a good sign that your insulin levels are low. This reflects a good state of insulin sensitivity, indicating you're ready to move to the Maintain stage.

PREVENT MEAL PLAN (15% CARBS)

	Breakfast	Lunch	Dinner
MONDAY	[Fasting]	Cobb Salad with Herb Ranch Dressing, page 146	Creamy Sun-Dried Tomato Chicken, page 158, and Soft Dinner Roll, page 210
TUESDAY	Strawberry Cheesecake Smoothie, page 125	leftover Creamy Sun-Dried Tomato Chicken, page 158, and Soft Dinner Roll, page 210	BBQ Pulled Pork Sliders, page 176, and Better-Than-Mashed-Potatoes, page 214
WEDNESDAY	Cheesy Sausage and Egg Casserole, page 132	leftover BBQ Pulled Pork Sliders, page 176, and Better-Than-Mashed-Potatoes, page 214	Hawaiian Meatballs and Spaghetti Squash Noodles, page 188
THURSDAY	[Fasting]	leftover Hawaiian Meatballs and Spaghetti Squash Noodles, page 188	Creamy Garlic Shrimp, page 194, and Favorite Noodles, page 218
FRIDAY	hard-boiled eggs and raw almonds	leftover Creamy Garlic Shrimp, page 194, and Favorite Noodles, page 218	Braised Lamb Shanks with Gravy, page 175, and The Best Broccoli, page 216
SATURDAY	Egg-Cheddar-Ham Sandwich, page 135	leftover Braised Lamb Shanks with Gravy, page 175, and The Best Broccoli, page 216	Smoky Spiced Brisket, page 184, and Spinach Salad with Bacon and Poppy Seed Dressing, page 145
SUNDAY	[Fasting]	leftover Smoky Spiced Brisket, page 184, and Spinach Salad with Bacon and Poppy Seed Dressing, page 145	Fall-Off-the-Bone Kimchi Pork Ribs, page 179, and Better-Than-Mashed-Potatoes, page 214

Notes: Begin and end each day with 2 tablespoons apple cider vinegar upon waking and before bed.

These meal plans are meant to be used simply as a suggestion, and portion sizes should be determined based on your overall caloric needs. While each dish may not fit the target carb count, the meal will hit the target when considering all of the dishes in combination.

10

Maintain

If you're on the Maintain track, you're a rare individual—among that 12 percent of adults who are insulin sensitive. You might have success if you simply keep doing what you're doing! However, given that so many begin descending the slippery metabolic slope to insulin resistance without being aware, there's value in viewing your current state as temporary. If you want to maintain your insulin sensitivity (and remember, that gets harder with age!), it's time to start making some shifts in your lifestyle to protect your health.

You have more freedom when it comes to your lifestyle habits. This is most obviously reflected in a higher portion of carbohydrates in the diet. Because you're insulin sensitive, eating a carbohydrate-heavy meal will have a much smaller effect on the amount of insulin secreted and, more importantly, on how long it remains elevated. Indeed, your insulin will likely be elevated less than half the time compared with someone eating the same foods but with underlying insulin resistance. But again, don't take this for granted—if you're spiking insulin too frequently, the insulin curve will steadily expand and before you know it, you've slipped down the slope. So there's still much benefit in eating to keep insulin low—and even fasting. While the sample meal plan that follows doesn't build in any fasts, revisit chapter 2 and challenge yourself to incorporate fasting into your weekly routine.

Exercise or engage in some kind of vigorous activity most days of the week. Whether this is a challenging walk (on the border of having to break into a run) or lifting weights (or your own body), make sure you're working hard. This is particularly important if you hope to gain and maintain muscle.

Remember, even if you're older, you can still significantly increase the size of your muscles by working them to exhaustion. Of course, the older we are, the more careful we want to be in pushing a joint too hard for fear of injury. Thankfully, the evidence suggests that even when doing more repetitions with a lighter weight, if the activity is performed to the point that the muscle is exhausted (that is, you can't do any more), you will have the same increase in muscle as if you used a heavier weight and performed fewer repetitions.

In the end, be vigilant. Throughout all of this, we come back to ketones. Don't forget the value in measuring ketones as a marker of insulin sensitivity. Testing ketones in the morning from time to time will be very helpful in letting you objectively measure your insulin-related status. Of course, measuring insulin resistance with various clinical tests described earlier is the best compass to ensure you're staying on track.

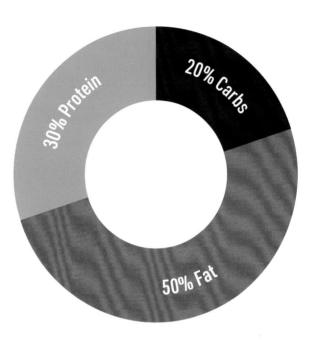

Maintain
Percent of Calories

20% Carbs

50% Fat

30% Protein

Time Your Carbohydrates

If your strategy includes more liberal amounts of carbohydrates, remember the "carbs come last" rule from chapter 5. When carbohydrates come after protein and fat, they are naturally digested more slowly. Not only does this lower what would be a higher insulin spike, but it actually even decreases the total time insulin is increased. Be careful not to abuse this, however. If you try to sneak refined carbohydrates in, with their naturally higher insulin spike, after eating very fatty foods, the combination of the high fat and insulin spike will be like fertilizer on your fat cells, both stimulating (via insulin) and fueling (via available fat in the blood) fat cell hypertrophy. So, if carbs are going to come last in your meal, focus on whole fruits and vegetables.

MAINTAIN MEAL PLAN (20% CARBS)

	Breakfast	Lunch	Dinner
MONDAY	Your New Favorite Breakfast Burrito, page 136 (or fasting)	Grilled Chicken Satay with Peanut Sauce, page 161, and avocado slices	Crispy Sweet Mongolian Beef, page 183, and Stir-Fried Rice, page 213
TUESDAY	Classic Omelet, page 139	leftover Crispy Sweet Mongolian Beef, page 183, and Stir-Fried Rice, page 213	Herb-Roasted Halibut, page 201, and Caramelized Peppers and Onion, page 215
WEDNESDAY	hard-boiled eggs, raw almonds, and berries (or fasting)	leftover Herb-Roasted Halibut, page 201, and Caramelized Peppers and Onion, page 215	Creamy Swedish Meatballs, page 187, and Better-Than-Mashed-Potatoes, page 214
THURSDAY	Cheesy Sausage and Egg Casserole, page 132	leftover Creamy Swedish Meatballs, page 187, and Better-Than-Mashed-Potatoes, page 214	Chicken Alfredo Spaghetti Bake, page 162, and Spinach Salad with Bacon and Poppy Seed Dressing, page 145
FRIDAY	Strawberry Cheesecake Smoothie, page 125 (or fasting)	leftover Chicken Alfredo Spaghetti Bake, page 162, and Spinach Salad with Bacon and Poppy Seed Dressing, page 145	Favorite Lamb Larb, page 172, and Favorite Noodles, page 218
SATURDAY	Baked Puffy Pancake, page 131	leftover Favorite Lamb Larb, page 172, and Favorite Noodles, page 218	Spiced Butter Chicken, page 157, and cauliflower rice
SUNDAY	Iced Apple Cinnamon Muffins, page 127 (or fasting)	leftover Spiced Butter Chicken, page 157, and cauliflower rice	Baja Fish Tacos, page 199, and The Best Broccoli, page 216

Notes: Begin and end each day with 2 tablespoons apple cider vinegar upon waking and before bed.

These meal plans are meant to be used simply as a suggestion, and portion sizes should be determined based on your overall caloric needs. While each dish may not fit the target carb count, the meal will hit the target when considering all of the dishes in combination.

Put It into Action

11

Before You Get Started

With all this knowledge now in your brain, it's just about time to put it into practice! Before we get there, though, we'd like to pause and talk strategy—some tactics that will help you embrace and adopt your new lifestyle with success. It may be helpful to stop thinking in terms of "healthy" or "not healthy" since *healthy* has become a watered-down word that means many different things to different people. Instead, it creates perfect clarity to aim for an *insulin-sensitive lifestyle*. Here are your new "golden rules":

* Don't fear fat! Wholesome fat is an excellent source of fuel that doesn't impact insulin.
* Avoid consuming carbohydrates before or after your workout, especially in the form of sugar. Your body doesn't need it, even after a tough workout.
* Intermittent and extended fasting is an excellent way to reduce excess body fat and to promote insulin sensitivity. (And fasting can be incredibly liberating!)

* Meat and dairy are excellent sources of fuel that don't impact insulin.
* Pay attention to reducing carbs rather than reducing calories, and simply eat until you are full.

While sculpted abs and a lean, athletic figure are a fantastic reward for living an insulin-sensitive lifestyle, the real benefit lies in improved overall health.

It will be easier than you think . . . but you're going to have to start with an open mind.

Your Mind Matters Most

The first step toward meaningful change is performed in the theater of your mind. Accomplishing a positive shift in your lifestyle requires that you see the new and improved version of yourself clearly in your mind long before it is physically reflected back at you in the mirror. What does the new version of you look like? How has your health improved? What kinds of foods does this new version of you eat? What is the new you's attitude toward exercise?

Not only is it beneficial to begin by spending time working on your mindset, it is a prerequisite for creating lasting improvement to your lifestyle, to your physical shape, and ultimately to your health. Don't get us wrong, anyone can white-knuckle a diet and fitness regime for a few weeks, but only those who are willing to do the initial mental and emotional groundwork will be rewarded with long-term success.

As Henry Ford wisely said, "Whether you believe you can do a thing or not, you are right." The importance of your own positive expectations cannot be overstated. It will determine your ultimate success. If it helps, know that we believe in you. But of course it's much more important that *you* believe in you.

Your Health Bank—Beware Insulin's Surcharge

You can think of every food you eat and every beverage you drink as a transaction in your "health bank." Every meal that contains little or no carbohydrates and instead prioritizes protein and healthy fat is a "deposit" that increases the available balance of your account, giving you resources and security. On the other hand, every meal containing more than 20% carbohydrates comes with an "insulin surcharge" that eats into your health fund. Periods of fasting that last 4 hours or longer are another positive deposit.

We all know how important it is to deposit more funds into our bank account than we withdraw. If you've ever overdrawn your bank account, you know how important it is to keep your finger on the ebb and flow of funds, erring on the side of excess rather than depletion. By stacking several deposits in your account, you know that it's OK to splurge and pay a surcharge every once in a while. However, if you continue to run up your account with carb-loaded transactions, don't be surprised when your health account becomes overdrawn.

Define Specific Goals

Having clarity on the improvements that you want to make with your health is like having a destination clearly marked on a map. You'll be able to measure whether you're getting closer to your goal and see when you start to get off track. It helps to have a big, **long-term goal** as well as many **short-term goals**. Imagine your long-term goal as being 100 miles away from you, and as you set out on foot to your ultimate destination, each mile marker along the way becomes a short-term goal to focus on. As long as you are constantly focused on reaching the next mile marker, you will surely end up at your ultimate destination in due time.

* In a journal or in the notes app on your phone, write out a description of your big, **long-term goal**. Example: *I will improve my metabolic health by reducing my waist circumference by 4 inches and my fasting glucose to 75 mg/dL.*

* Next, write out several **short-term goals** to help you toward your long-term goal. Example: *This week I will exercise 4 times, fast between meals, and keep all meals except dinner free from carbs.*

* Update your **long-term goal** every so often, as you make progress. The picture that you have of your vision for yourself will constantly evolve and become clearer with each day that you work toward it. This is a good thing! Take the time to write it out and spend mental energy thinking about it each day.

* Congratulate yourself for every **short-term goal** achieved. A quiet moment when you feel the significance of your achievement and allow yourself to feel satisfaction, accomplishment, and confidence will go far in training your brain to keep on winning. As soon as each short-term goal has been achieved, set your sights on the next one and start working toward it.

Modify Your Habits

Most of us are creatures of habit, even if not all of our habits were created intentionally. Habits make life smooth and reduce the number of decisions that we must make each day. For instance, there are usually a handful of things that you eat for breakfast. You have your go-to lunch and snacks that rarely change. Dinners rotate through familiar homemade or ordered-in meals. While this can work against us when our lifestyle is insulin-spiking, it's a beautiful thing once insulin-sensitizing habits become our mainstays.

As you go through a review of your typical day, you might be surprised how many things you do out of habit! Once you've identified the habits that are working against your efforts to improve your health, it's as simple as finding a healthier alternative to insert into its place.

In a journal or in the notes app on your phone, write out what you typically eat for breakfast, lunch, snacks, dinner, and after dinner. Highlight the items that need to change. Now spend some time coming up with insulin-sensitizing alternatives. Here are some examples:

	Your Old Habit	Your New Habit
Breakfast	Bagel with scrambled egg	Scrambled egg with avocado
Lunch	Sandwich, chips, and a cookie	Salad, almonds, and berries
Snack	Coffee shop pastry	Iced tea sweetened with stevia
Dinner	Burrito, rice, and beans	Easy Chicken Enchilada Casserole (page 165) and cauliflower rice

Next, think about the restaurants that you frequent. Jot down your typical order; if you're seeing a big carb load, pull up the restaurant menus and come up with a new order that falls in line with your goals. Keep this list handy for the inevitable moment in the future when you find yourself ordering from these menus. Here are some examples:

* Burger or sandwich place: Order your favorite burger or sandwich wrapped in lettuce or served over salad.
* Italian place: Swap out the pasta in your favorite dish for steamed broccoli.
* Mexican place: Have the meat from your favorite tacos served in a bowl with shredded lettuce, salsa, sour cream, and pico de gallo.
* Pizza place: Get a salad with your favorite pizza toppings tossed into it—or make Meatzza Pizza, page 153, at home!

Transform Your Kitchen

It's time to raid your kitchen—it is probably filled with insulin-spiking foods that need to be removed from the premises! Take a bag or box and go through your pantry, cupboards, fridge, and freezer, collecting everything that you know will get you off track. Make your best judgment on which should be given away or donated and which need to end up in the trash or compost.

Once that's done, it's time to go shopping for insulin-sensitive replacements for everything you just got rid of.

Schedule Your Workouts

Exercise really doesn't do much if you do it only once in a blue moon. The real benefits to strengthening and conditioning your body are found in consistency. That doesn't mean that you must exercise every single day, but you certainly should 3 or 4 times per week.

Whether you're planning to use the workouts in this book, or do your own thing, first pull out your calendar and block off your workout times. Not only will this serve as a constant reminder, it will reinforce your commitment to taking this proactive step toward better health. The next chapter will walk you through a workout if you don't already have an exercise routine.

If you have the resources and availability to join a boot camp–style group exercise program or work directly with a fitness trainer, pick up the phone and schedule your first session. Do it now! The environment will guarantee your adherence and success in getting your exercise done because of the accountability, expertise, consistency, variety, and support:

- **Accountability:** Having a fitness coach and exercise buddies waiting for you to show up makes a world of difference when your internal resistance starts to kick in, which it is guaranteed to do at some point. Accountability is priceless.
- **Expertise:** Working with a trained coach will ensure not only that you are performing each exercise correctly, but that you're pushing yourself hard enough to reap the most rewards.

- **Consistency:** When you work with a professional, or are part of an exercise group, your workouts get scheduled into your calendar (and your phone blows up with texts and calls when you miss a day).
- **Variety:** Another huge benefit to working with a professional or joining a boot camp–style gym is the variety of movements that will be thrown your way. The next chapter lays out solid foundational moves, but it's always a good thing to keep your body guessing by changing things up often.
- **Support:** There will be days, or even seasons, of your life when you need real, human support in your fitness journey. An injury. An illness. A bout of boredom with your routine. A vacation that gets you out of the habit permanently. You name it, there will be many times along the way where you'll benefit from the support of a real, human coach and a community to lift you up.

Lastly, a comment about the expense. As the saying goes, *you value what you pay for.* Free, or super low cost, sounds great, but in the end you'll take something seriously when you invest your hard-earned money into it. Money spent on your physical fitness by working with a professional fitness coach in your area is a priceless investment.

Stay Strong (and Tap Your Support System)

What happens when you're sitting down to lunch with your coworkers and your meal looks a lot different than theirs? Or when the office is celebrating a colleague's birthday with slices of cake? Or when your family gathering revolves around traditional, nostalgic foods that you know will lead to a big insulin spike?

Look, you could easily slide back into old habits, but you wouldn't have gotten this far in the book if you weren't pretty determined already to make some changes in your life. The people in your life who have your best interests at heart are going to applaud your new lifestyle . . . and they might even be drawn in by your positive example to make insulin-sensitizing changes of their own. (The positive ripple effect that takes place when you make positive changes in your life is one of the sweetest rewards. So if you feel weak in the face of peer pressure, think about doing it for those you love most.)

Communicate your intentions with the important people in your life. It's understandable if you're hesitant to make any big announcements, especially if you've made attempts to improve your health in the past that didn't stick. However, the power of a support system is worth a few moments of vulnerability. Talk with your significant other, your immediate family, and the friends with whom you regularly spend time. Let the important people in your life know that you are making some big changes to your lifestyle in order to achieve better health, longevity, and quality of life, and directly ask for their support.

People outside your inner circle don't need to be looped in, although don't be surprised when they start to notice the changes in you as you make progress. Be concise and definitive when sharing the news of your evolving lifestyle. Let them know your goal, your health-based reason for the goal, and the changes that they will be seeing in your habits. Then ask that they please support your efforts. Direct and open communication like this is a great way to create your very own network of support to give you a hand when you need it most.

The Power of Consistent Small Measures

Every day we are given the opportunity to make dozens and dozens of decisions. What to eat, where to go, what to say, what to do . . . each moment brings us multiple choices. While it is unrealistic to expect yourself to make the best, healthiest, most optimal decision at every minute, you can seek out small, feasible measures as a way of life.

No positive effort is ever too small to matter.

If you don't have time for a full workout today, could you do 10 squats or a minute of jumping jacks? If you simply must have that burger, could you ditch half of the bun? Could you stand instead of sitting at work this afternoon? Could you take the stairs instead of the elevator? Could you refrain from having seconds at dinner?

Moving toward a more insulin-sensitizing lifestyle doesn't have to be undertaken in giant leaps. Baby steps can get you there too. The key is to keep striving and to keep your eye on the prize. You've got this!

12

Let's Move

The goal for this chapter is to wipe away all of the confusion and complications and reduce exercise down to its simplest and most doable forms. A plan that won't intimidate or confuse you. One that you might even enjoy!

In chapter 6, we described exercise as "a period of time wherein the muscles engage in repetitive and exhausting movement." It really doesn't have to be any more complicated than that! Your job in each workout is to push your body out of its resting state into a rapidly moving, exerting state with a simple list of compound movements and high-intensity intervals. It will be simple. And fun! We promise.

Note, if you are currently doing a fitness routine that includes challenging, regular exercise sessions several times a week, then please pat yourself on the back and move on to the next chapter. You're already doing what you need! As long as your consistent exercise routine includes both resistance training and cardiovascular exercise with sufficient intensity, then you are good to go.

What Equipment Do I Need?

You don't need a gym membership or fancy equipment to meet your exercise needs each week—only your body. While working with a fitness coach or group can be a great resource (as discussed in chapter 11), if that is simply not an option for you and you have zero equipment at your disposal, you can easily use the body weight exercises in the following pages for a perfectly adequate exercise regime. A sturdy chair can help you balance and act as a supportive surface for certain moves.

If you're looking to add some equipment to your arsenal, exercise bands, such as the ones shown in the following photos, are inexpensive and a great investment. Exercise bands are extremely versatile and are great for creating resistance against which your muscles can work.

The next tier of equipment would be a pair or two of dumbbells, an exercise ball, and finally a barbell. The exercises in this chapter can be modified to use these for greater results.

Beginner Resistance Exercises

The following exercises are a great place to start if you are a beginner to exercise, or if it has been a while since you have maintained a consistent exercise routine. These movements have been modified to reduce the load as you begin to strengthen muscles and build endurance. The number of repetitions or reps that you do will depend upon the person and how much weight you're using; perform to exhaustion (8 to 20 reps usually does the trick). Once these exercises begin to feel less challenging, simply move on to the more challenging exercises that follow.

Squat to Chair: Stand with your back to a chair, with your feet shoulder width apart, your back straight, and your arms straight out in front of you. Inhale as you bend at the knees, being careful not to extend your knees past your toes, dropping until your glutes touch the chair and your knees are at a 90-degree angle. Exhale as you rise back up to the starting position.

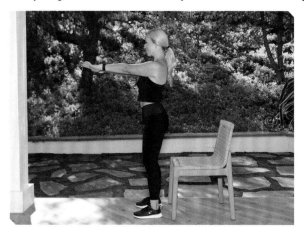 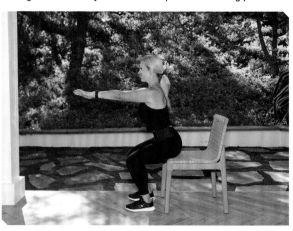

Lunge with Chair: Stand behind a chair with your feet together, your back straight, and your hands on the back of the chair. Inhale as you take a large step back and bend your back knee, being careful not to lean forward or extend your front knee past your toes, dropping until your front thigh is parallel to the ground and your front knee is at a 90-degree angle. Exhale and grip the chair for support as you push back up through your heel, returning your foot to the starting position. Repeat on the other side.

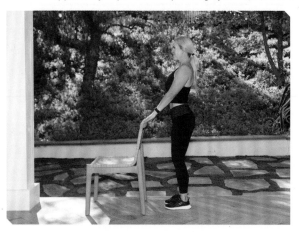 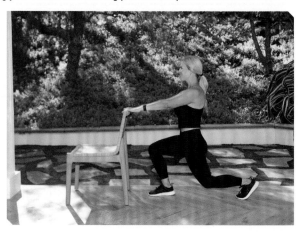

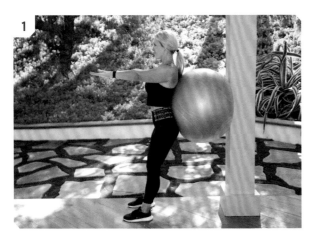

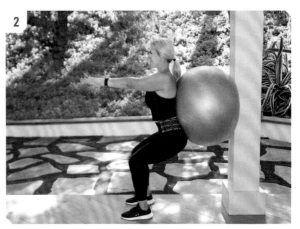

Ball Wall Sit: Position an exercise ball against the wall and press your upper back into it. Stretch your arms out in front of you. Slide down into a squat position until your knees reach a 90-degree angle. Keep your back pressed into the exercise ball and pull in your belly button. Hold for 30 to 60 seconds. If you don't have an exercise ball, simply perform this exercise by pressing your back directly into the wall.

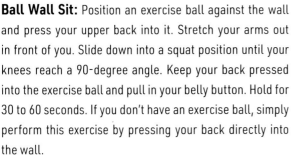

Modified Push-Up: Place your hands on the back of a chair (or against a countertop or wall) and assume a push-up position with your feet shoulder width apart. Keeping your back flat, inhale as you bend your elbows back and lower your body toward the ground. Exhale as you press back up to the starting position.

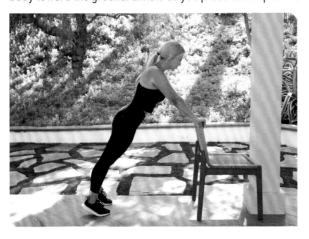

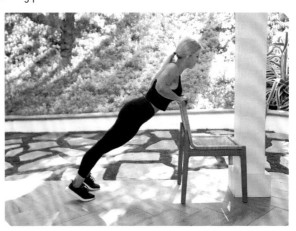

Knee Push-Up: On your hands and knees, assume a push-up position with your knees shoulder width apart and your palms on the floor below your shoulders. Keeping your back flat, inhale as you bend your elbows back and lower your body toward the ground. Exhale as you press back up to the starting position.

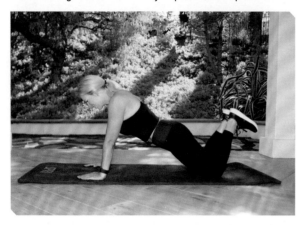 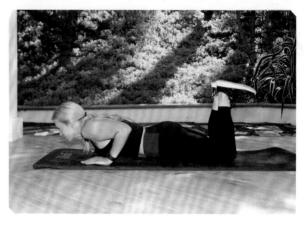

Modified Mountain Climber: Place your hands on a sturdy stool (or the bottom step of the stairs) and assume a push-up position with your feet shoulder width apart and palms elevated. Keeping your back flat, inhale as you alternate driving your knees in toward your chest.

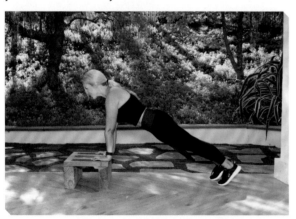 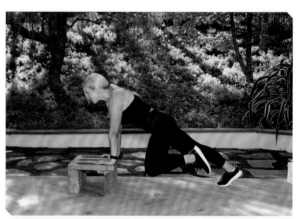

Modified Plank: On your elbows and knees, assume a push-up position with your knees shoulder width apart, your elbows and forearms pressed into the floor, and your ankles crossed. Keeping your back flat and a 90-degree angle in your elbows, focus on keeping your belly button pulled in toward your spine. Rather than a number of reps, hold the plank to exhaustion (as you get more experienced, up the challenge—and have fun!—by timing your plank and seeing if you can build up to longer and longer plank hold times, and move on to regular planks rather than modifying).

>>

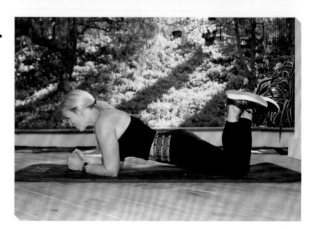

Here is a library of resistance exercises, using body weight and up through the various pieces of equipment mentioned earlier. Here we are focusing on compound movements that utilize multiple muscles at a time to increase the efficiency and effectiveness of your workout. Again, the number of repetitions or reps that you do will depend upon your experience level and how much weight you're using; perform to exhaustion (8 to 20 reps usually does the trick).

Squat Curl to Overhead Press: Stand with your feet shoulder width apart, your back straight, and your arms at your sides, gripping a band, dumbbells, or a barbell in your hands. Inhale as you bend at the knees, being careful not to extend your knees past your toes, dropping until your thighs are parallel to the ground and your knees are at a 90-degree angle. Exhale as you rise back up to the starting position, curling your fists up to your shoulders. Once in a standing position, extend your arms straight up, over your head. Inhale as you return your arms to the starting position.

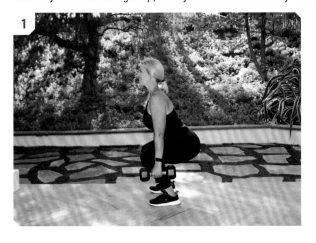

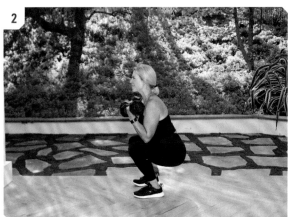

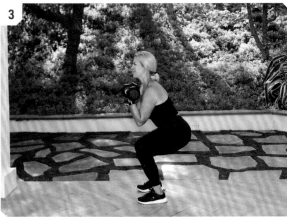

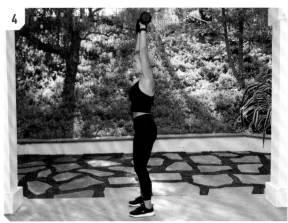

Squat: Stand with your feet shoulder width apart, your back straight, and your arms straight out in front of you. Inhale as you bend at the knees, being careful not to extend your knees past your toes, dropping until your thighs are parallel to the ground and your knees are at a 90-degree angle. Exhale as you rise back up to the starting position.

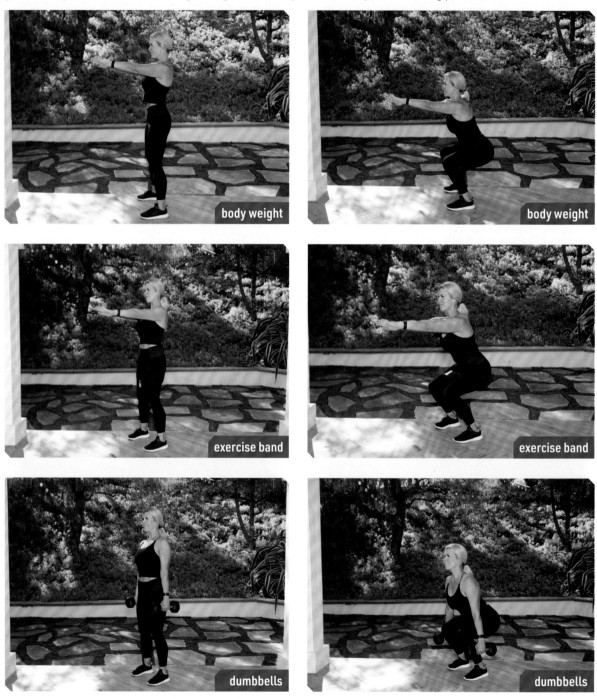

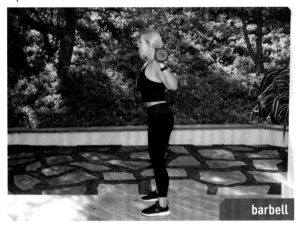

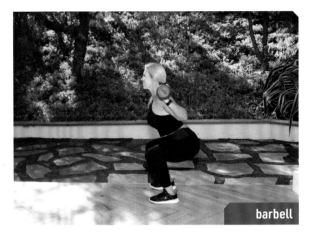

Split Squat: Stand with feet in a split stance, with your front heel 2 feet in front of your back foot and your back straight. Inhale as you bend at the knees, being careful not to lean forward or to extend your knees past your toes, dropping until your front thigh is parallel to the ground and your front knee is at a 90-degree angle. Exhale as you rise back up to the starting position. Repeat on the other side.

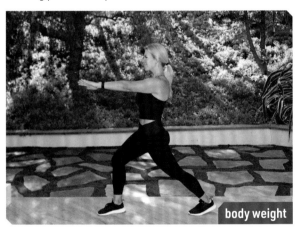

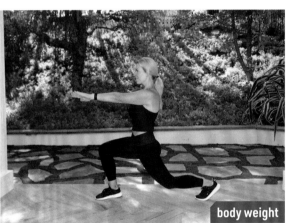

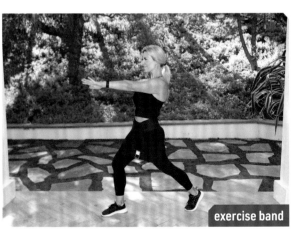

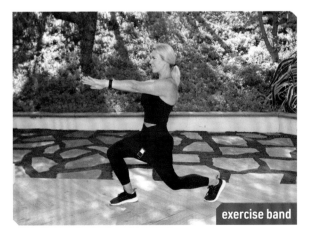

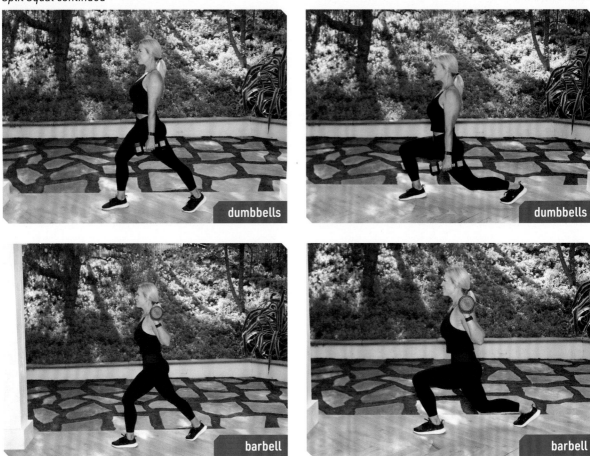

Lunge: Stand with feet together and your back straight. Inhale as you take a large step forward and bend your front knee, being careful not to lean forward or to extend your knees past your toes, dropping until your front thigh is parallel to the ground and your front knee is at a 90-degree angle. Exhale as you push back up through your front heel, returning your foot to the starting position. Repeat on the other side.

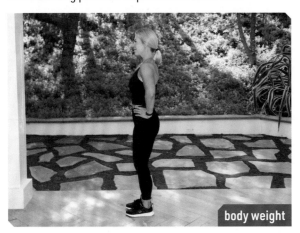

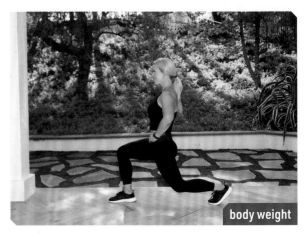

Lunge continued

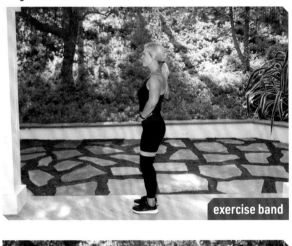

exercise band

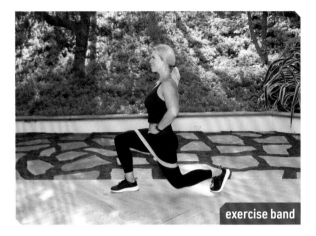

exercise band

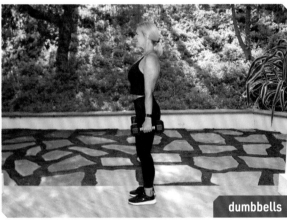

dumbbells

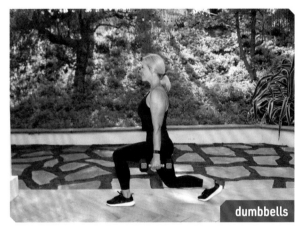

dumbbells

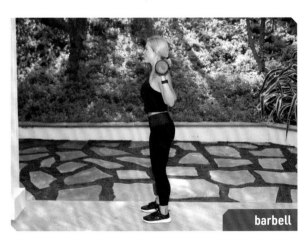

barbell

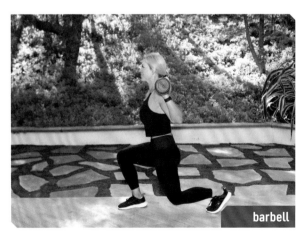

barbell

Squat to Pull-Apart: Stand with your feet shoulder width apart, your back straight, and your arms straight out in front of you, gripping a band or dumbbells. Inhale as you bend at the knees, being careful not to extend your knees past your toes, dropping until your thighs are parallel to the ground and your knees are at a 90-degree angle. Exhale as you pull the band or dumbbells apart and out to your sides, then rise back up to the starting position. Once in a standing position, inhale as you slowly bring your arms back together in front of your body.

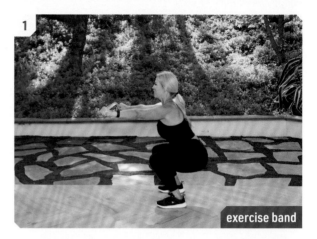

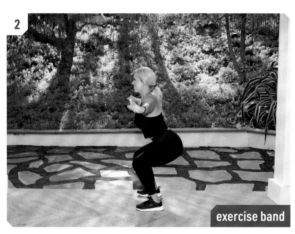

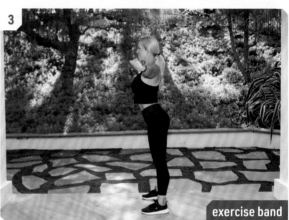

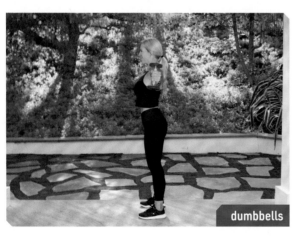

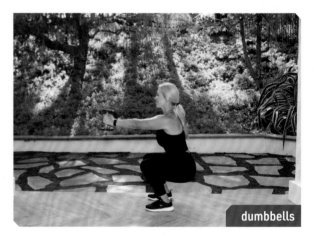

Deadlift: Stand with your feet shoulder width apart and your back straight. Inhale as you bend at the waist, keeping your back flat and allowing a slight bend in your knees, dropping your chest down until your back is parallel to the ground. Exhale as you straighten back up, squeezing your back and glutes as you return to the starting position.

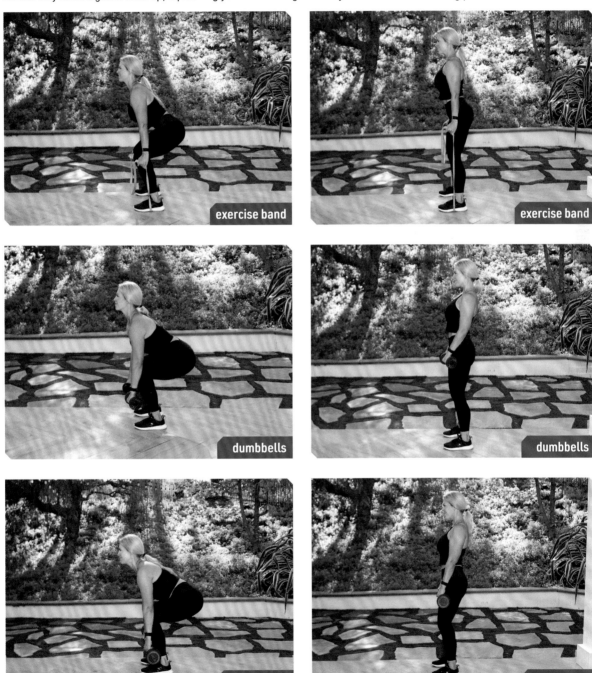

Chest Press: Lie with your upper back securely against an exercise ball or on the floor, with your feet shoulder width apart, feet securely on the ground and knees bent at a 90-degree angle. Keep your glutes elevated so that your body is in a straight line. Grip dumbbells, an exercise band, or a barbell in your hands above your chest. Exhale as you press the weight up above your chest, straightening your elbows and squeezing your chest and glutes. Inhale as you slowly return to the starting position.

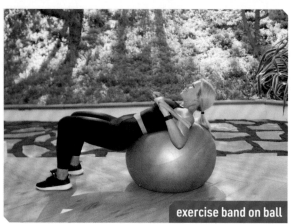
exercise band on ball

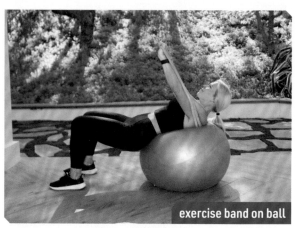
exercise band on ball

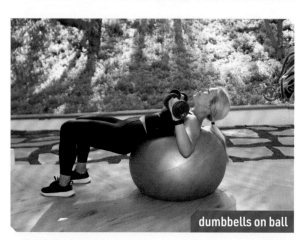
dumbbells on ball

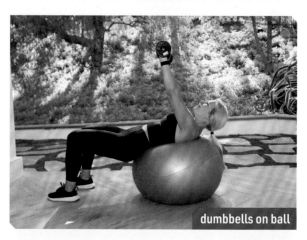
dumbbells on ball

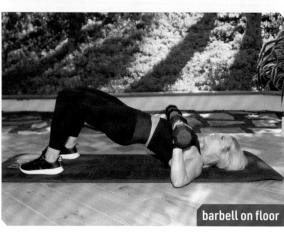
barbell on floor

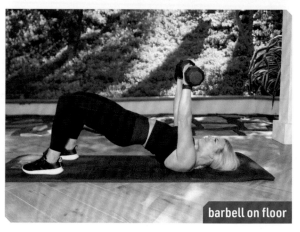
barbell on floor

Bent-Over Row: Stand with your feet shoulder width apart and a slight bend in your knees. Bend forward at the waist, keeping your back flat. Grip dumbbells, an exercise band, or a barbell in your hands, allowing it to hang down in front of your shins. Exhale as you bend your elbows back and draw your fists in toward your belly button, while squeezing your shoulder blades together. Inhale as you return to the starting position. For single-arm dumbbell rows, use the back of a chair for support as needed.

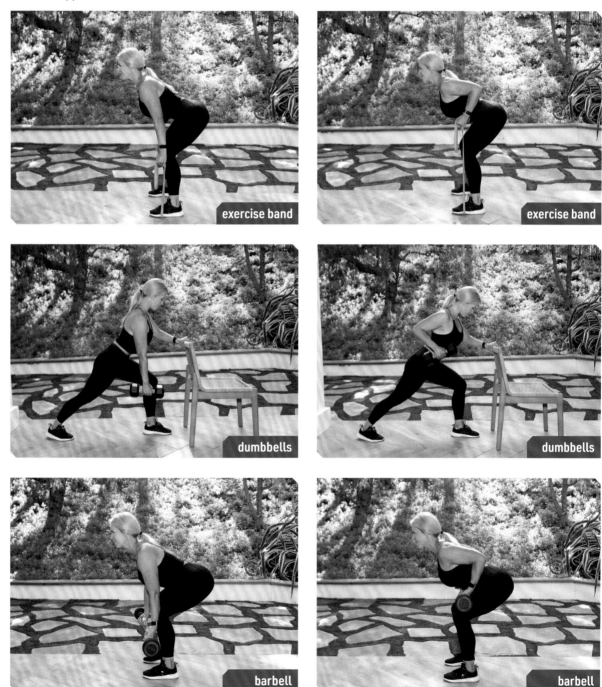

Slow Side Shuffle: Standing with your feet shoulder width apart, drop down to a 45-degree bend in your knees with your back flat and shoulders back. Maintain this position as you take a slow, deliberate 1-foot step to the right with your right foot, followed by a slow, deliberate 1-foot step to the right by your left foot. Continue for 8–20 steps before changing direction and moving to the left, back to the starting position.

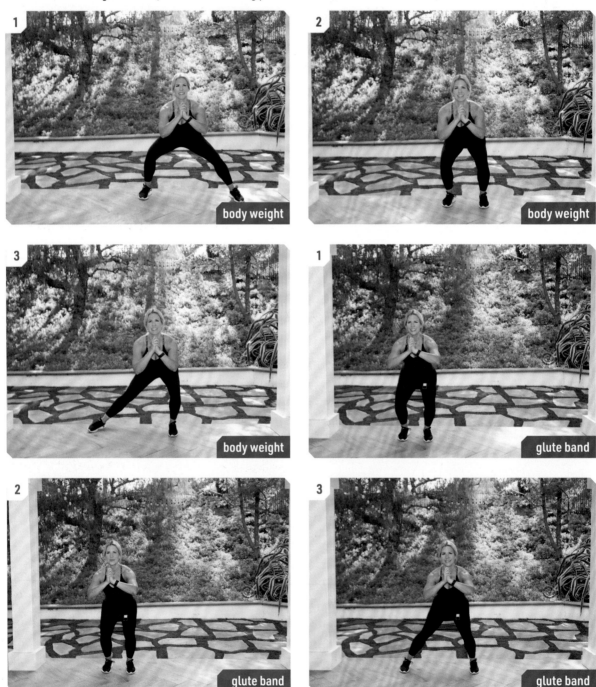

Dip: Place your palms behind you on the edge of a chair. Press your heels into the ground in front of you, feet shoulder width apart and a 90-degree angle in your knees. Inhale as you bend your elbows back, lowering your body down until your elbows reach a 90-degree angle. Keep your stomach and legs tight as you exhale and return to the starting position.

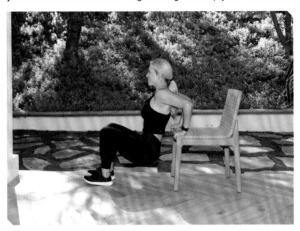 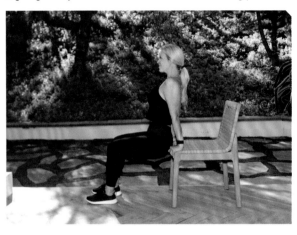

Push-Up: Assume a push-up position with your feet shoulder width apart and your palms on the floor below your shoulders. Keeping your back flat, inhale as you bend your elbows back and lower your body toward the ground. Exhale as you press back up to the starting position.

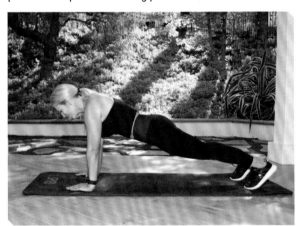 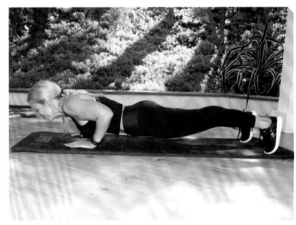

Pike Push-Up: Assume a push-up position with your feet shoulder width apart and your palms on the floor below your shoulders. Walk your feet in and push your glutes into the air to form an upside-down V. Keeping your back flat, inhale as you bend your elbows and lower your head toward the ground. Exhale as you press back up to the starting position.

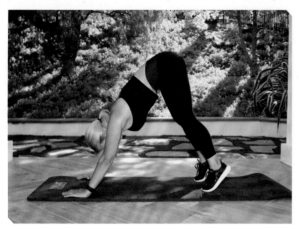 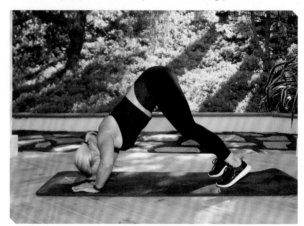

Wall Sit: Press your upper back into a wall and slide down into a squat position until your knees reach a 90-degree angle. Keep your back flat against the wall and pull in your belly button. Hold for 30 to 60 seconds. >>

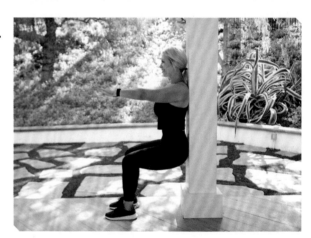

Core Exercises

There's more to your core than just your abdominal muscles—and working out your core is key to a well-rounded movement plan. Core exercises strengthen your hips, pelvis, lower back, and stomach, which can help you improve your balance and stability (lowering the risk of falls), mitigate lower back pain, and make it easier for you to do other movements.

Toe Touch: Lie on your back with your legs straight up in the air. Exhale as you extend your arms and reach toward your toes, keeping your back flat and legs straight. Inhale as you slowly return to the starting position.

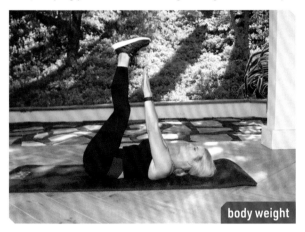

body weight

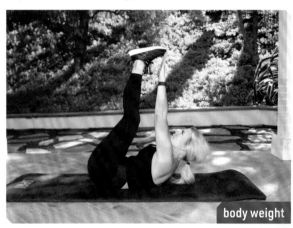

body weight

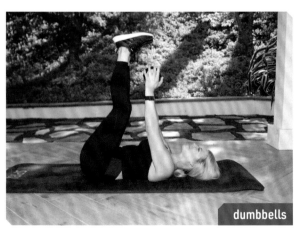

dumbbells

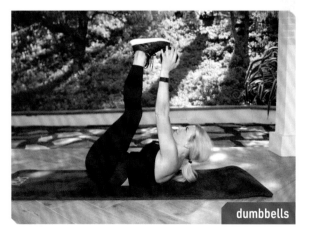

dumbbells

Flutter Kick: Lie flat on your back with your hands beneath your glutes. Exhale as you lift your feet off the ground, keeping your legs extended with a slight bend in your knees. Alternate flutter-kicking your feet up and down about a foot while keeping your abdominals tight and ensuring your back is pressed flat against the floor.

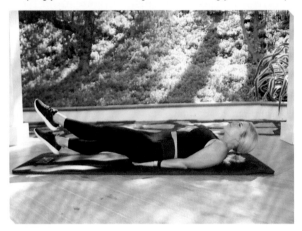 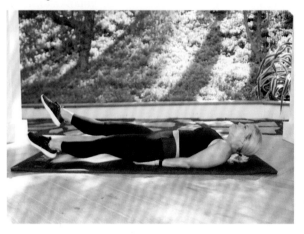

Side Reach: Lie on your back with your feet flat on the ground and your knees bent. Exhale as you lift your back off the ground, keeping it flat and hinging at your waist. Alternate reaching toward each ankle.

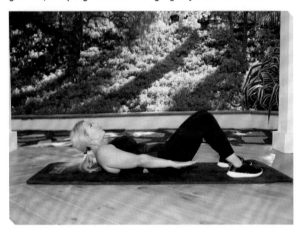 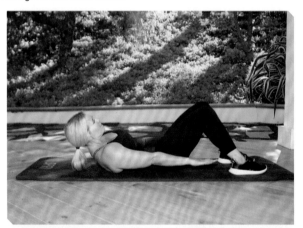

Hollow Hold: Lie on your back with your arms at your side. Exhale as you lift your legs and back off the ground in a V shape, reaching toward your ankles. Hold for 15 to 20 seconds.

>>

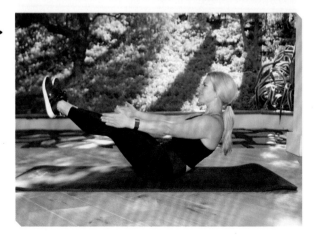

Plank: Assume a push-up position, with your feet shoulder width apart, toes anchored into the ground and your elbows and forearms pressed into the ground. Keeping your back flat and a 90-degree angle in your elbows, focus on pulling your belly button in toward your spine. Hold the plank to exhaustion (as you get more experienced, up the challenge—and have fun!—by timing your plank and seeing if you can build up to longer and longer plank hold times).

>>

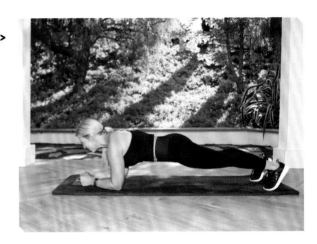

Glute Bridge: Lie on your back with your feet flat on the ground, knees bent, and arms at your sides. Exhale as you press your heels into the ground and lift your hips into the air, squeezing your glutes and pulling your belly button in toward your spine. Hold at the top for 5 to 10 seconds.

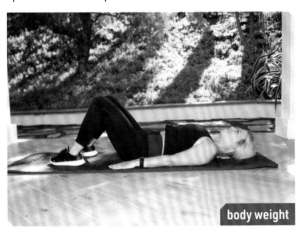

body weight

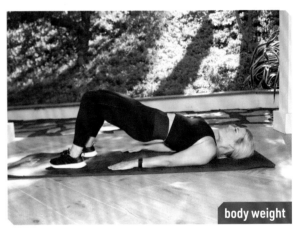

body weight

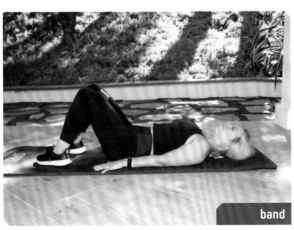

band

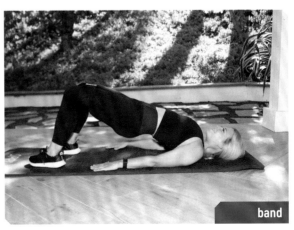

band

Crunch: Lie on your back with your feet flat on the ground and knees bent, hands behind your neck and elbows out. Exhale as you lift your upper back off the ground, bringing your chest straight up toward the ceiling, hinging at your waist and keeping your back flat. Inhale as you slowly return to the starting position.

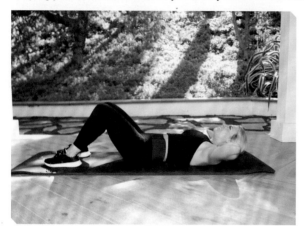

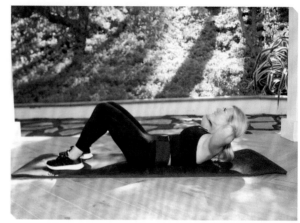

Dead Bug: Lie on your back with your feet off the ground, your knees bent at a 90-degree angle, and your arms straight up in the air. Inhale as you simultaneously lower your left arm above your head while straightening and lowering your right leg toward the ground. Switch sides and continue for 30 seconds.

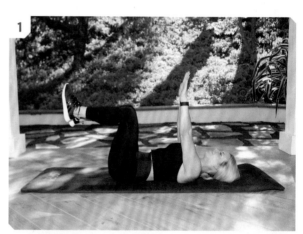

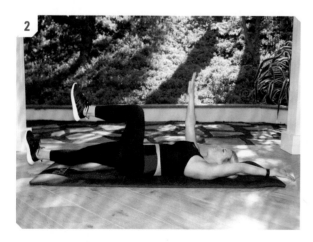

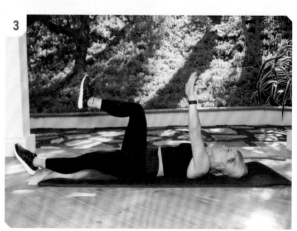

Russian Twist: Sit on the ground with your legs stretched out in front of you and a slight bend in your knees. Lift your feet up off the ground while keeping your shoulders back and back flat. Twist your upper body from side to side while keeping your feet off the floor and pulling your belly button in toward your spine.

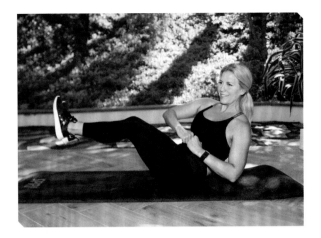

Standing Side Crunch: Stand with your feet shoulder width apart and hands near your ears with elbows out. Exhale as you lift your left knee toward your left elbow, crunching your left side and pausing at the top of the movement to squeeze your abdominals. Inhale as you return your foot to the ground and repeat on the other side.

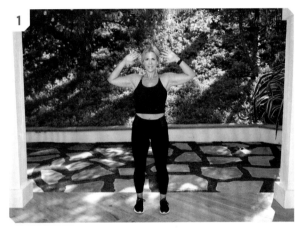

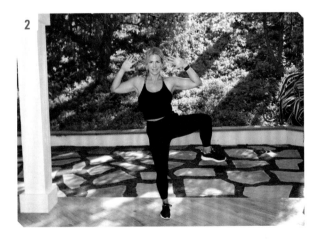

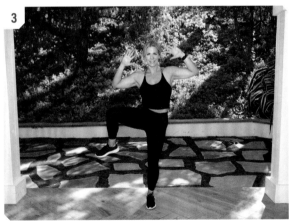

Dumbbell Side Crunch: Stand with your feet shoulder width apart and a slight bend in your knees. Place your right hand on your waist and hold a dumbbell in your left hand with your arm hanging down at your side. Exhale as you lean toward the left, squeezing your left side as the dumbbell reaches for your knee. Inhale as you straighten back up to the starting position. Repeat on the other side.

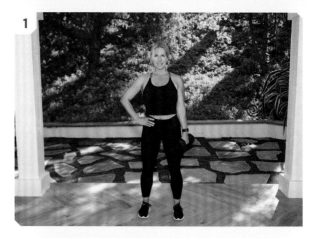

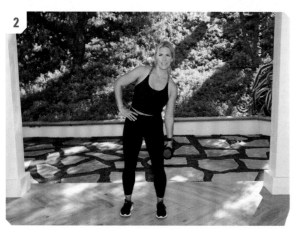

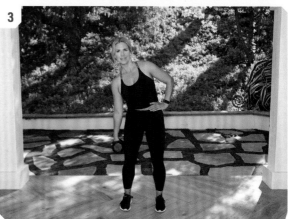

Superman: Lie on your stomach with your arms outstretched in front of you and eyes facing the ground. Exhale as you lift your arms and legs up while squeezing your glutes and back. Hold for 15 to 30 seconds before returning to the starting position.

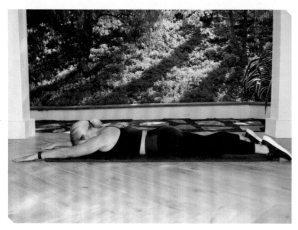

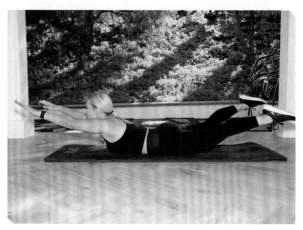

Aerobic Exercises

These aerobic exercises use body weight and up through the various pieces of equipment mentioned, organized from easier to more advanced moves. We are focusing on high intensity and movements that utilize multiple muscles at a time, increasing the efficiency and effectiveness of your workout. Do what's safe for your body. Additionally you could run, walk, hike, bike, swim, dance, or utilize cardio equipment (such as an elliptical machine).

Burpee: Assume a push-up position with your feet shoulder width apart and palms on the ground below your shoulders. Keeping your back flat, inhale as you bring your knees in toward your chest, pressing your feet together and your heels into the ground. Exhale as you jump straight up in the air, with your arms stretched above your head, then land lightly in heel-toe order. Return to the starting position and repeat to exhaustion.

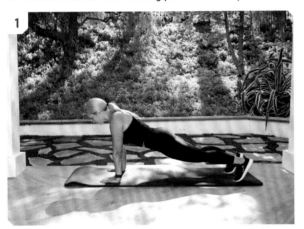

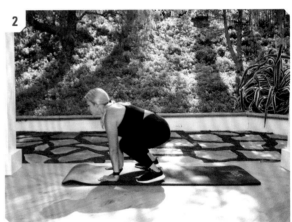

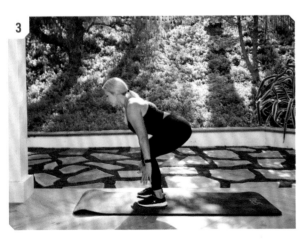

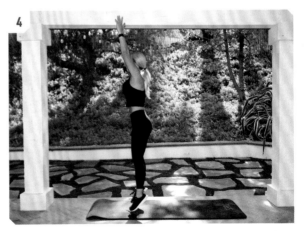

Standing March: Stand with your feet shoulder width apart and a slight bend in your knees. Lift your left foot off the ground until your thigh is parallel to the ground and there is a 90-degree bend in your knee, keeping your right foot firmly planted into the ground and swinging your right elbow forward in an exaggerated marching movement. Return your left foot to the ground as you switch to the opposite arm and leg.

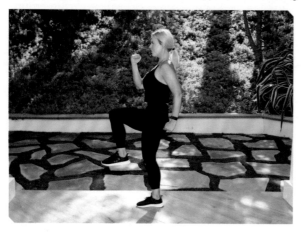
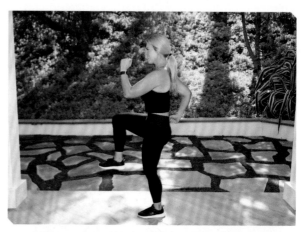

High Knees: Stand with feet shoulder width apart, back straight, and arms straight in front of you with palms facing down. Alternate lifting your knees up to touch your palms as quickly as you can. Repeat to exhaustion.

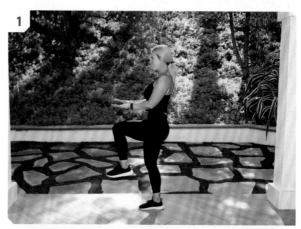

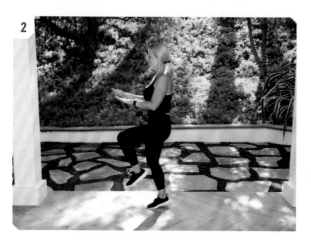
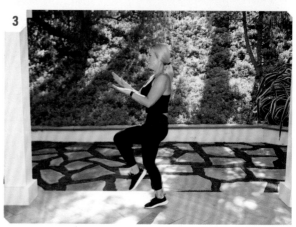

Jumping Jack: Stand with feet together, back straight, and arms down at your sides. Inhale as you jump, your feet apart and hands together over your head. Exhale as you lower your arms back to your sides and jump your feet back together. Repeat to exhaustion.

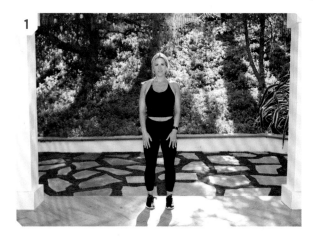

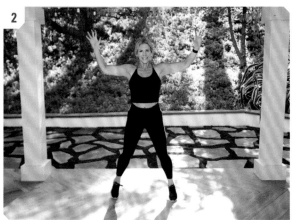

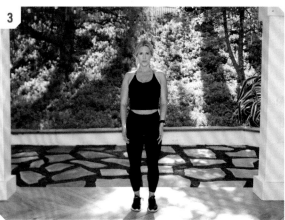

Jump Squat: Stand with feet shoulder width apart and your back straight. Inhale as you bend at the knees, being careful not to extend your knees past your toes, dropping until your thighs are parallel to the ground and your knees are at a 90-degree angle. Exhale as you jump straight up in the air, then land lightly in heel-toe order. Repeat to exhaustion.

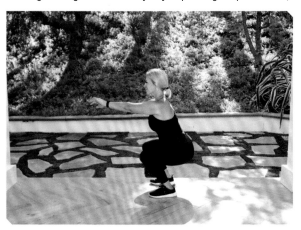

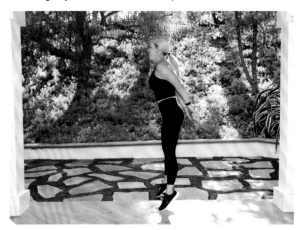

Step-Up: Stand in front of a sturdy stool (or the bottom step of the stairs) with your feet shoulder width apart and a slight bend in your knees. Step onto the stool with your left foot and lift your right knee up in the air. Return your left foot to the ground as you switch to the other side.

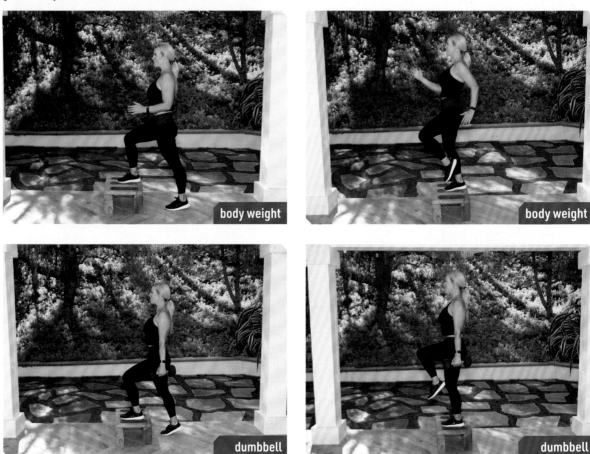

Hill Sprint: On your mark, get set, go! Run as fast as you can for 30 to 90 seconds, up a hill if you have one, otherwise increase the running time to 3 minutes on a flat surface.

Jump Rope: Stand with your feet shoulder width apart and a slight bend in your knees. Jump as you swing the jump rope over your head and underneath your feet.

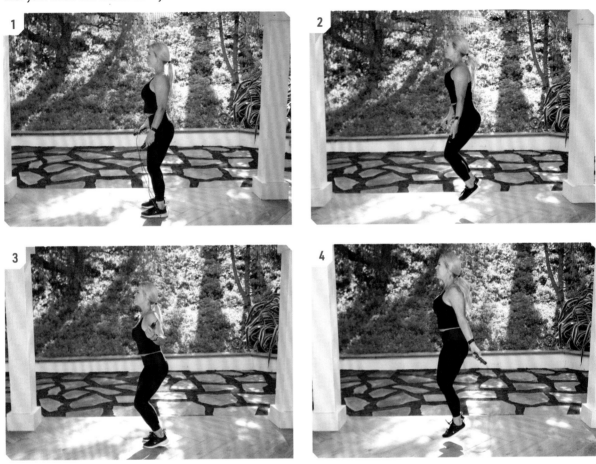

Mountain Climber: Assume a push-up position with your feet shoulder width apart and palms flat on the floor. Keeping your back flat, inhale as you alternate driving your knees in toward your chest.

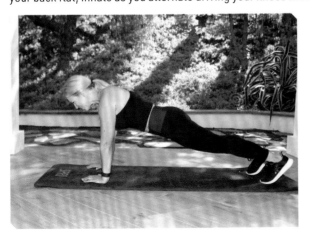 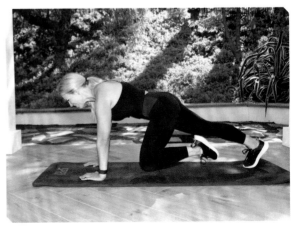

Sample Workouts

6-Minute Abs

Here's the only ab routine you'll ever need! Perform this 6-minute routine after your main workout, while you're still warm, otherwise take a few moments to warm up with some walking beforehand.

There are plenty of ways to keep it interesting, and it's just long enough to smoke your abs without feeling too strenuous. It's broken up into 8 segments of 45 seconds, so set your smartphone to beep every 45 seconds for 8 rounds. If you know other ab exercises, feel free to utilize different exercises in between the rounds of flutter kicks.

Round 1: 45 seconds	Flutter Kicks
Round 2: 45 seconds	Crunches
Round 3: 45 seconds	Flutter Kicks
Round 4: 45 seconds	Toe Touches
Round 5: 45 seconds	Flutter Kicks
Round 6: 45 seconds	Plank
Round 7: 45 seconds	Flutter Kicks
Round 8: 45 seconds	Side Reaches

Simple Shred Burn

In this simple workout, we shred with our resistance exercise and burn with the aerobic. Before beginning your shred burn workout, do some light stretching, walking, or jogging to get warmed up.

Choose one resistance exercise and one aerobic exercise from the preceding library. Perform the resistance exercise to exhaustion. Take 30 to 90 seconds to recover, then move swiftly into the aerobic exercise, performing it vigorously until exhaustion. Take another 30 to 90 seconds to recover before repeating both exercises again. Repeat this for 5 sets (5 times doing each exercise) before entering a cool-down period of walking and stretching. That's it! Change up the exercises that you choose often, to keep your body guessing and all of your muscles working, and feel free to add additional sets as you build up your stamina.

10 Shred Burn Workouts

Squat Curl to Overhead Press	+	Hill Sprints
Lunges	+	Mountain Climbers
Deadlifts	+	Jumping Jacks
Push-Ups	+	Jump Squats
Bent-Over Rows	+	Jump Rope
Body Weight Dips	+	Hill Sprints
Slow Side Shuffle	+	Jumping Jacks
Chest Press	+	Jump Squats
Squat to Pull-Aparts	+	Jump Rope
Split Squat	+	Step-Ups or Burpees

Circuit Workouts for the Week

Here is a sample week of workouts for different levels of fitness. It is important that you build your strength and endurance by increasing the resistance and intensity of your workouts gradually rather than starting out too hard. It is also important that you progressively challenge yourself as you become more conditioned, rather than sticking with what feels comfortable.

This workout plan is to be performed as a circuit. Start with exercise #1 and perform 15 to 30 repetitions or 30 to 60 seconds. Rest for 30 seconds and then move on to exercise #2. After completing one set of each exercise, perform the aerobic exercise for 1 to 5 minutes. Repeat the circuit until you've completed the target number of rounds: 3 rounds for Beginner, 4 rounds for Intermediate, and 5 rounds for Advanced.

> **Your job in each workout is to push your body out of its resting state into a rapidly moving, exerting state with a simple list of compound movements and high-intensity intervals. It will be simple. And fun! We promise.**

Beginner Weekly Exercise: 3 Rounds

	Exercise #1	Exercise #2	Aerobic
Monday	Squat to Chair	Modified Push-Up	Standing March
Tuesday	REST	REST	REST
Wednesday	Dips	Lunge with Chair	Modified Mountain Climber
Thursday	REST	REST	REST
Friday	Slow Side Shuffle	Bent-Over Row	Step-Ups
Saturday	Ball Wall Sit	Chest Press	Walking
Sunday	REST	REST	REST

Intermediate Weekly Exercise: 4 Rounds

	Exercise #1	Exercise #2	Exercise #3	Aerobic
Monday	Squat with dumbbell	Bent-Over Row	Flutter Kick	Jumping Jacks
Tuesday	Push-Up	Superman	Squat to Pull-Apart	Jump Rope
Wednesday	Slow Side Shuffle with band	Dips	Plank	High Knees
Thursday	REST	REST	REST	REST
Friday	Lunge with dumbbell	Deadlift	Squat Curl to Overhead Press	Step-Up with dumbbell
Saturday	Russian Twist	Wall Sit	Dead Bug	Mountain Climbers
Sunday	REST	REST	REST	REST

Advanced Weekly Exercise: 5 Rounds

	Exercise #1	Exercise #2	Exercise #3	Exercise #4	Aerobic
Monday	Split Squat with barbell	Standing Side Crunch with dumbbell	Push-Up	Hollow Hold	Jump Squat
Tuesday	Side Reach	Slow Side Shuffle with band	Pike Push-Up	Glute Bridge with band	Hill Sprint
Wednesday	Bent-Over Row	Flutter Kick	Lunge with dumbbell	Plank	Burpee
Thursday	Chest Press	Dips	Russian Twist	Squat with band	Jump Rope
Friday	Squat Curl to Overhead Press	Dead Bug	Crunch	Deadlift	High Knees
Saturday	Push-Up	Squat to Pull-Apart	Toe Touch with dumbbell	Bent-Over Row	Step-Up with dumbbell
Sunday	REST	REST	REST	REST	REST

Carb-Conscious Recipes

13

It's time to get cooking! In this chapter, you'll find 72 delicious carb-conscious recipes to help you keep insulin low.

We want to acknowledge that food is not just fuel for most of us. Food is habit. Food is comfort. Food is tradition. Food is nostalgic. Food is so intertwined with love that it can be difficult to separate the two. This emotional layer to food adds complexity when a well-meaning scientist and lifestyle coach come along and ask you to change how you eat. (Honestly, how dare we!?) But, as we've outlined in the previous chapters, something must change to ensure your best body and health. And that something is the food that you were likely raised on and may have been eating for decades.

That said, let us reassure you that this does *not* mean a life of tasteless, boring, unappetizing meals. Not on Diana's watch! As you'll see in the upcoming pages, cooking for insulin sensitivity can be downright mouthwatering.

These recipes mostly use ingredients that likely will be familiar to you (like wholesome dairy and eggs, meat and seafood, and fresh veggies). There are just a few specialized ingredients you might need to add to your arsenal:

- Almond flour
- Coconut flour
- Coconut aminos
- Swerve or other brand of erythritol (granular, brown, and confectioners)

Recipes to Reverse, Prevent, and Maintain

Each of the following recipes fits in with one or more of the insulin-sensitizing plans outlined earlier in the book. Look for the icons on each:

R These recipes are suitable for the Reverse phase and can also be enjoyed on the Prevent and Maintain tracks.

P These recipes are great if you are on the Prevent or Maintain track.

M There are fewest of these because these recipes have relatively higher net carbs and are suitable only for those on the Maintain track.

Strawberry Cheesecake Smoothie ⓡ ⓟ ⓜ

Per serving: Calories: 339 Fat: 21g Net Carb: 7g (8%) Protein: 26g
Makes 1 serving | **Prep time: 5 minutes**

Combine all of the ingredients (except the optional topping) in a blender. Blend until smooth. Pour into a glass, top with whipped cream if desired, and enjoy immediately.

2 tablespoons heavy cream
1 cup water
1 ounce cream cheese
1 scoop sugar-free vanilla or strawberry protein powder
1 tablespoon granular Swerve
½ cup ice
½ cup frozen strawberries
Sweet Whipped Cream (page 230) or sugar-free whipped cream, for topping (optional)

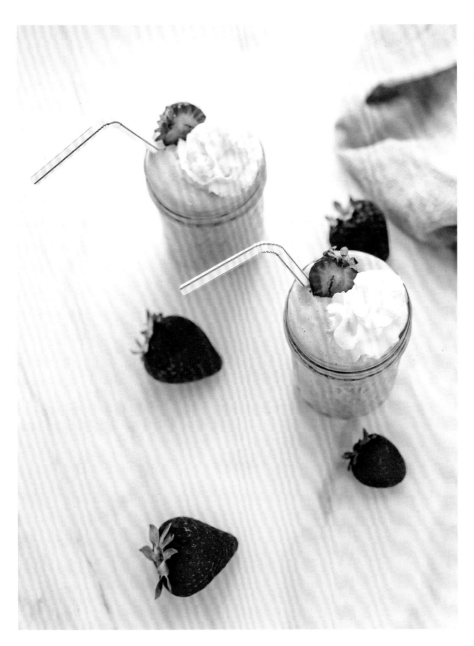

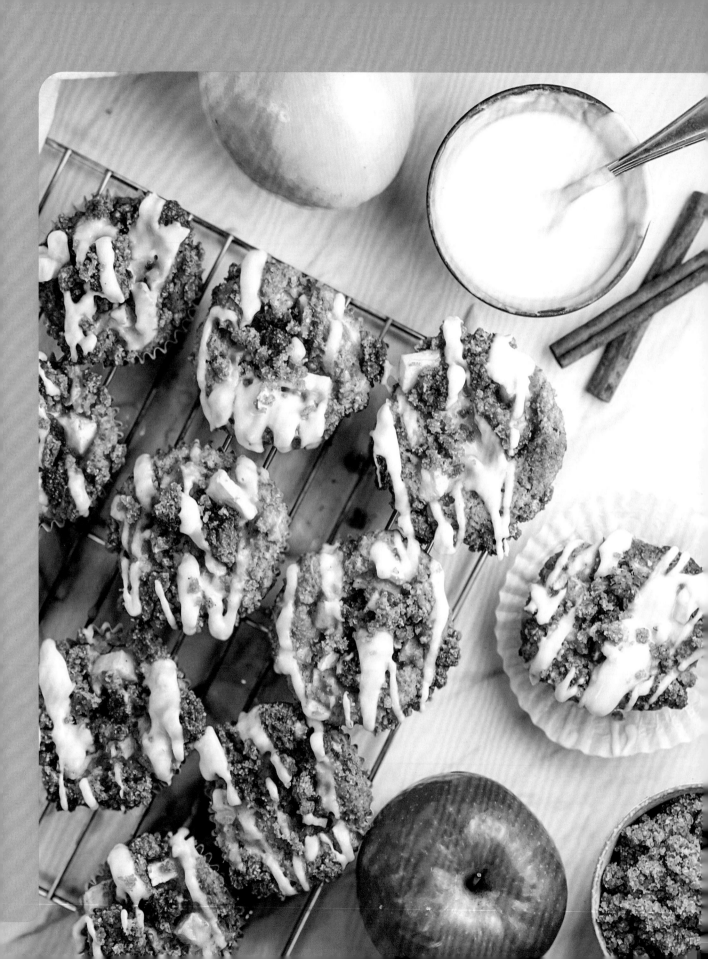

Iced Apple Cinnamon Muffins Ⓟ Ⓜ

Per muffin: Calories: 208 Fat: 17g Net Carb: 6g (11%) Protein: 8g
Makes 12 muffins | **Prep time: 25 minutes** | **Cook time: 20 minutes**

Preheat the oven to 425 degrees F. Line a muffin tin with 12 paper or silicone liners. Set aside.

In a mixing bowl, whisk together the almond flour, coconut flour, baking powder, baking soda, salt, and cinnamon to remove any lumps; set aside.

Pour about an inch of water into a small saucepan and bring to a simmer. Put the mozzarella cheese in a heatproof bowl and set it on top of the saucepan, making sure the bottom of the bowl does not touch the water below. Stir the mozzarella until fully melted, then remove the bowl and let cool slightly. Add the sour cream, eggs, brown Swerve, granular Swerve, and vanilla and mix until well combined. Stir in the dry ingredients. Fold in the apple until just combined. Divide the batter evenly among the 12 muffin cups.

Combine all of the crumb topping ingredients in a small bowl; the mixture should be crumbly. Sprinkle the topping over the tops of the muffins.

Bake for 5 minutes, then reduce the oven temperature to 350 degrees F. Bake for an additional 15 minutes, or until the muffins are golden on the outside and fully set. Remove from the oven and let cool on a wire rack.

While the muffins bake, combine the vanilla icing ingredients in a small bowl. Drizzle over the cooled muffins.

Muffins
- 1 cup almond flour
- ¼ cup coconut flour
- 1 teaspoon baking powder
- 1 teaspoon baking soda
- ¼ teaspoon salt
- 1 teaspoon ground cinnamon
- 2 cups shredded mozzarella cheese
- ¼ cup full-fat sour cream
- 2 large eggs
- ⅓ cup brown Swerve
- ¼ cup granular Swerve
- 2 teaspoons vanilla extract
- ¾ cup chopped peeled apple

Crumb Topping
- ⅓ cup brown Swerve
- 1 tablespoon granular Swerve
- 1 teaspoon ground cinnamon
- 4 tablespoons (½ stick) unsalted butter, melted
- ⅔ cup almond flour

Vanilla Icing
- 1 cup confectioners Swerve
- 3 tablespoons heavy cream
- ½ teaspoon vanilla extract

Tip: Have some fun by changing up the flavors of your muffins. Blueberry: Swap out the chopped apple for ⅔ cup blueberries. Jalapeño Cheese: Omit the brown Swerve and reduce the granular Swerve to 2 tablespoons, swap the chopped apple for a 4-ounce can of diced green chiles (drained), and swap out the icing and crumb topping for 1 pickled jalapeño (finely chopped) and a sprinkle of cheddar cheese. Chocolate Chip: Swap out the chopped apple for 1 cup stevia-sweetened chocolate chips.

Fluffy Pancakes ⓡ ⓟ ⓜ

Per serving: Calories: 390 Fat: 34g Net Carb: 5g (5%) Protein: 14g
Makes 4 servings | **Prep time: 10 minutes** | **Cook time: 15 minutes**

1½ cups almond flour
1 teaspoon baking powder
1 tablespoon granular
    Swerve
¼ teaspoon salt
3 large eggs
⅓ cup heavy cream
¼ teaspoon vanilla extract
1 tablespoon unsalted butter,
    melted, plus more for
    greasing (optional)
Sliced fresh fruit or berries,
    for serving (optional)
Zero-sugar syrup, for serving
    (optional)

Preheat a griddle or large skillet over medium-high heat. In a mixing bowl, whisk together the almond flour, baking powder, Swerve, salt, eggs, heavy cream, and vanilla. Stir in the melted butter until well combined.

Grease the griddle with additional butter or coconut oil. Reduce the heat to low. Working in batches as necessary, use a ¼ cup measure to scoop the batter onto the griddle, leaving space between the pancakes. When bubbles form (after 2–3 minutes), flip the pancakes to cook on the other side, 2–3 minutes more.

Serve with fresh fruit and a drizzle of syrup if desired.

Tip: There are many zero-sugar syrups available to replace traditional, insulin-spiking maple syrup. Look for ones sweetened with natural, zero-sugar sweeteners like stevia, monk fruit, or erythritol.

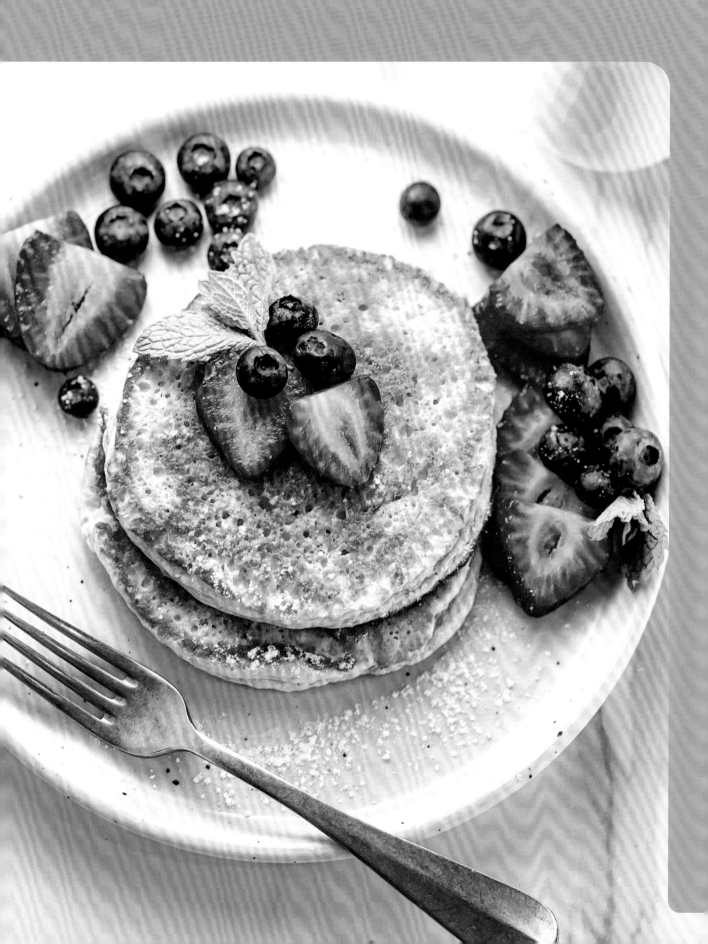

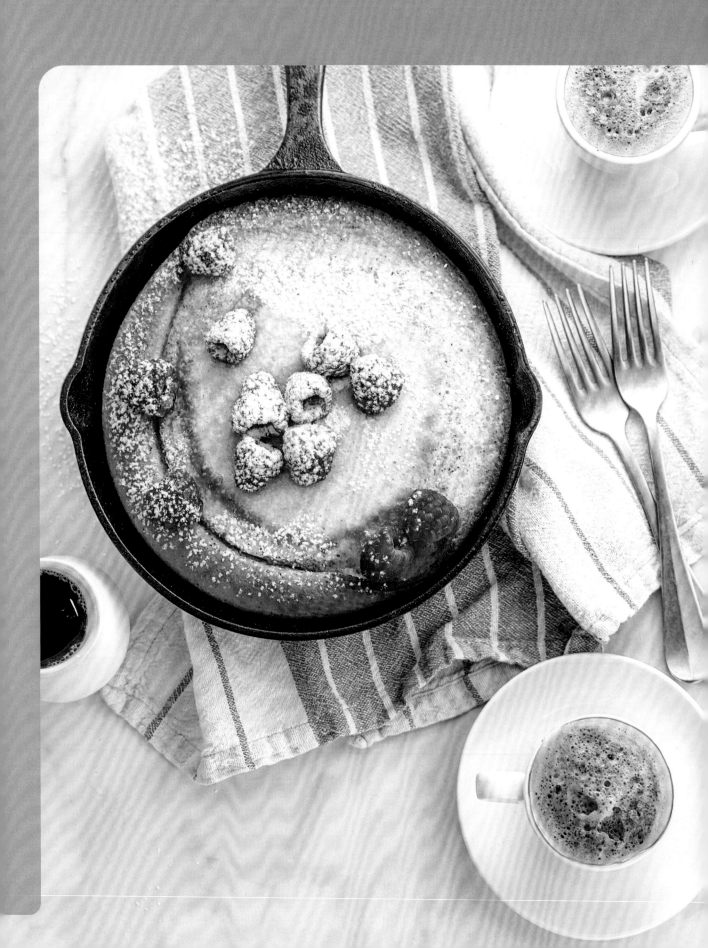

Baked Puffy Pancake 🅡 🅟 🅜

Per serving: Calories: 281 Fat: 27g Net Carb: 4g (6%) Protein: 5g
Makes 4 servings | **Prep time: 10 minutes** | **Cook time: 20 minutes**

Preheat the oven to 425 degrees F. Place an 8-inch cast-iron skillet in the oven while it preheats.

In a food processor, blend the eggs, heavy cream, sour cream, and 1 tablespoon of melted butter. Add the almond flour, coconut flour, baking powder, salt, granular Swerve, vanilla, and lemon zest. Blend until smooth, scraping down the sides as needed.

Using pot holders, remove the hot skillet from the oven. Being careful to hold the skillet away from you, add 2 tablespoons of butter to the skillet and swirl to coat the entire bottom. The butter may spatter.

Pour the batter into the skillet and return it to the oven. Bake for 10 to 15 minutes, until there is no longer any jiggling in the center of the pancake. Turn on the broiler and cook for 5 minutes, until the top is golden. Remove the skillet from the oven and immediately brush the pancake with the remaining 1 tablespoon of melted butter. If desired, top with confectioners Swerve and a handful of raspberries, then cut into 4 wedges and drizzle with syrup.

3 large eggs
¼ cup heavy cream
¼ cup full-fat sour cream
4 tablespoons (½ stick) unsalted butter, melted, divided
½ cup almond flour
2 tablespoons coconut flour
1 teaspoon baking powder
¼ teaspoon salt
3 tablespoons granular Swerve
1½ teaspoons vanilla extract
½ teaspoon grated lemon zest
Confectioners Swerve, for serving (optional)
Fresh raspberries, for serving (optional)
Zero-sugar syrup, for serving (optional)

Cheesy Sausage and Egg Casserole Ⓡ Ⓟ Ⓜ

Per serving: Calories: 307 Fat: 25g Net Carb: 2g (3%) Protein: 18g
Makes 8 servings | **Prep time: 15 minutes** | **Cook time: 30 minutes**

8 large eggs
¼ cup heavy cream
½ teaspoon salt
¼ teaspoon black pepper
1 cup shredded Colby jack cheese, divided
1 tablespoon unsalted butter
1 tablespoon minced garlic
1 pound ground pork sausage
½ cup diced green bell pepper
½ cup diced red bell pepper
4 green onions, chopped
Magic Sauce (page 135), for serving (optional)

Preheat the oven to 400 degrees F. Grease a 9-inch baking pan with butter.

In a large mixing bowl, whisk together the eggs, cream, salt, and pepper until fully combined. Mix in ½ cup of cheese. Set aside.

Melt the butter in a medium skillet over medium-high heat. Add the garlic and cook until fragrant, about 2 minutes. Add the sausage and cook, breaking it up with a wooden spoon, until browned, about 5 minutes. Add the bell peppers and green onions and cook until the vegetables are soft, about 3 minutes.

Transfer the contents to the prepared baking pan and spread into an even layer. Pour the egg mixture over the sausage mixture. Sprinkle the remaining ½ cup of cheese over the top.

Bake for 25 minutes, or until cooked through and golden. Cool for 10 minutes, then slice and serve, with sauce if desired.

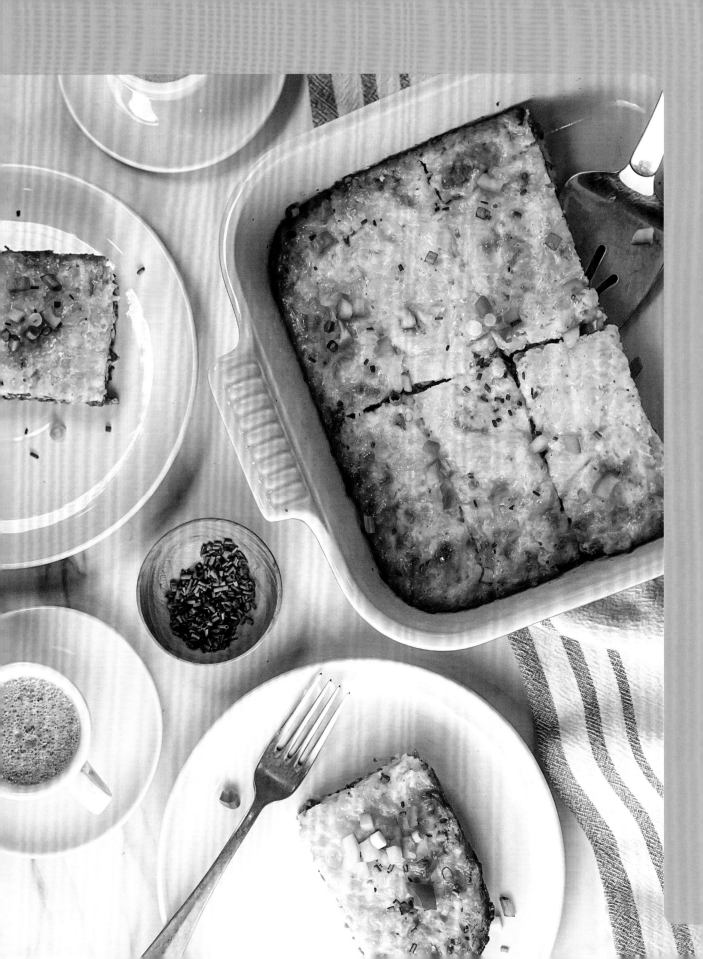

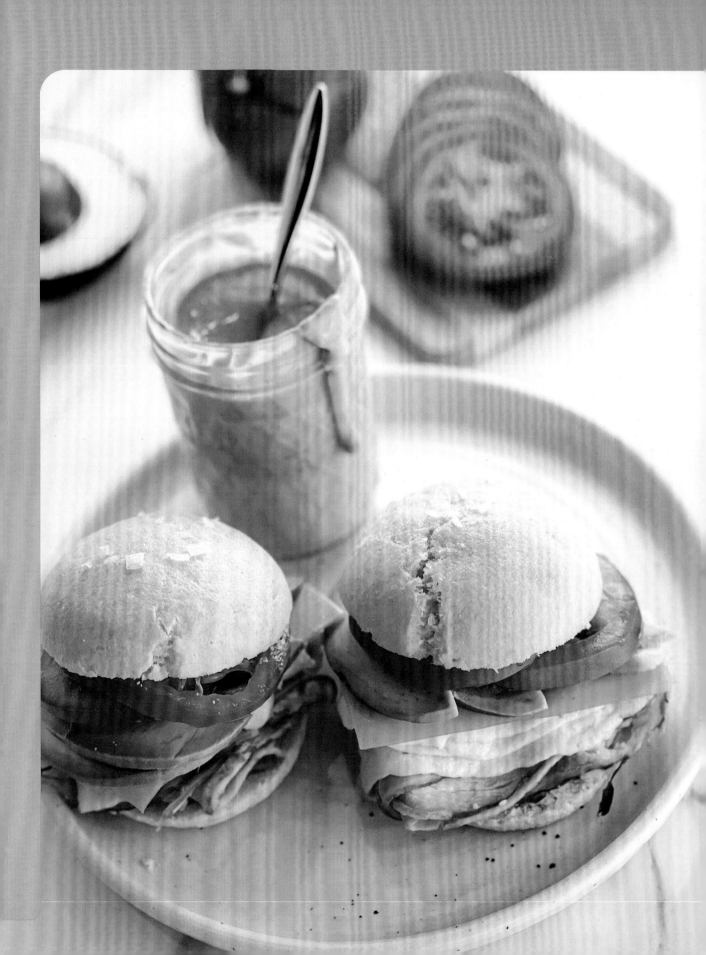

Egg-Cheddar-Ham Sandwich Ⓡ Ⓟ Ⓜ

Per serving: Calories: 493 Fat: 39g Net Carb: 7g (6%) Protein: 34g
Makes 1 serving | **Prep time: 5 minutes** | **Cook time: 5 minutes**

In a small bowl, whisk together the egg and cream. Heat a small nonstick skillet over medium-low heat. Add the egg mixture and cook, undisturbed, until set, about 2 minutes. Use a spatula to flip the egg and cook the other side for 10 seconds. Transfer the egg to a plate or cutting board and fold it in half, then in half again.

In another small bowl, whisk the sauce ingredients together until smooth.

Spread the bottom half of the roll with a bit of sauce. (Store leftover sauce in an airtight container in the fridge for up to 2 weeks.) Stack the ham, egg, cheese, tomato, and avocado on top. Place the top half of the roll on the stack and enjoy immediately.

Sandwich
1 large egg
1 tablespoon heavy cream
1 Soft Dinner Roll (page 210), sliced in half
1 slice ham
1 slice cheddar cheese
2 slices tomato
¼ avocado, sliced

Magic Sauce
¼ cup full-fat sour cream
1 teaspoon yellow mustard
1 tablespoon no-sugar-added BBQ sauce
1 tablespoon brown Swerve
Pinch salt

Your New Favorite Breakfast Burrito Ⓡ Ⓟ Ⓜ

Per serving: Calories: 318 Fat: 26g Net Carb: 8g (10%) Protein: 15g
Makes 2 servings | **Prep time: 15 minutes** | **Cook time: 5 minutes**

Egg Tortillas
2 large eggs
1 teaspoon heavy cream
1 teaspoon coconut flour
⅛ teaspoon onion powder
Pinch salt
Pinch black pepper
1 tablespoon unsalted butter
¼ cup shredded cheddar
   cheese

Burrito Filling
½ avocado
Dash lime juice
Pinch salt
1 tablespoon pico de gallo
¼ cup cooked crumbled
   sausage
½ cup shredded drained
   zucchini
1 tablespoon minced green
   onion

In a small bowl, whisk together the eggs, cream, coconut flour, onion powder, salt, and pepper until smooth.

Melt the butter in a medium skillet over medium-low heat, swirling to evenly coat the bottom. Pour the tortilla batter into the skillet. Cook, undisturbed, until bubbles form in the center of the tortilla, about 3 minutes. Use a spatula to loosen the sides of the tortilla. Flip the tortilla and sprinkle with the cheddar cheese. Cook for an additional 10 seconds. Transfer the tortilla to a plate.

In another small bowl, mash the avocado with a squeeze of lime juice and a pinch of salt.

Spread the avocado mixture over the tortilla. Spoon the pico de gallo, ground sausage, shredded zucchini, and green onion in a line down the middle of the tortilla. Roll the tortilla over the filling, slice in half, and serve immediately.

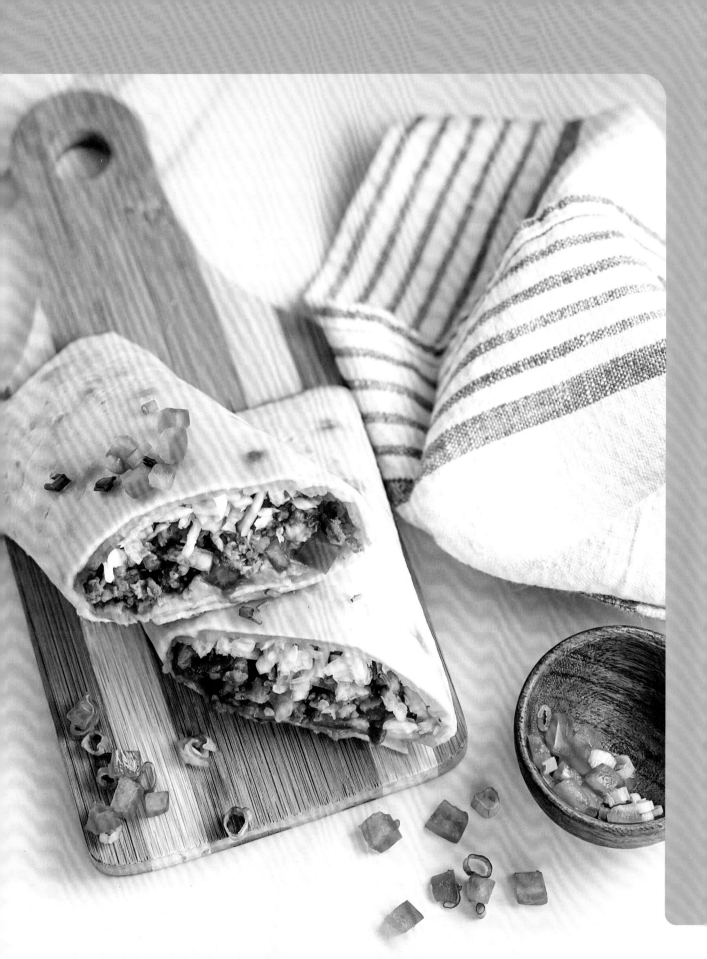

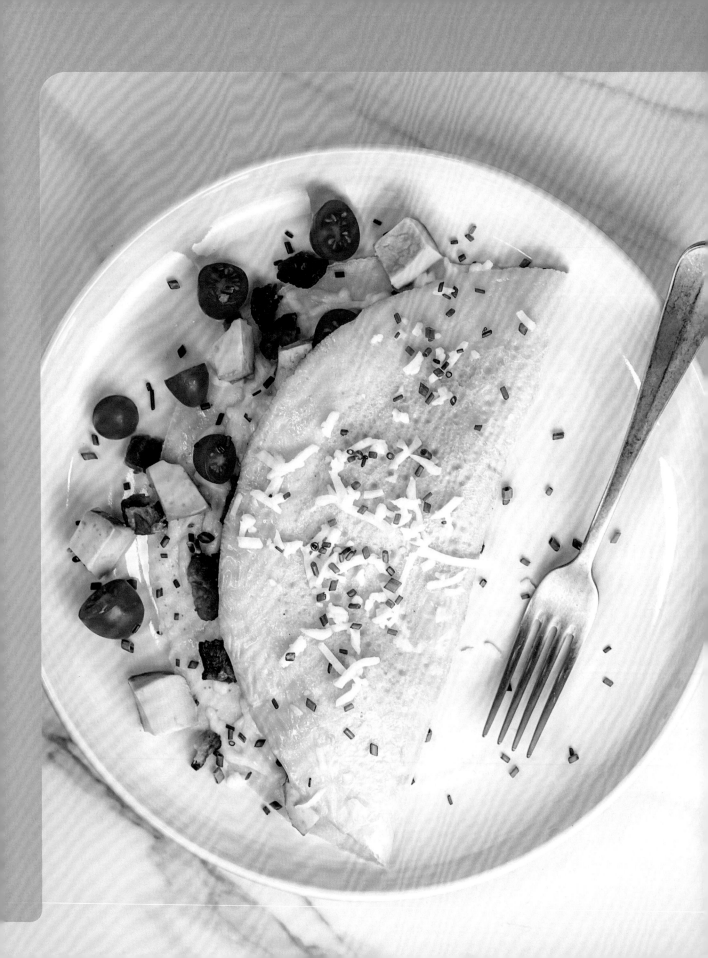

Classic Omelet ⓡ ⓟ ⓜ

Per serving: Calories: 460 Fat: 32g Net Carb: 9g (8%) Protein: 31g
Makes 1 serving | Prep time: 10 minutes | Cook time: 5 minutes

Coat a small skillet with cooking spray and heat over medium heat. Add the mushrooms and sauté until lightly browned, about 4 minutes. Using a slotted spoon, transfer the mushrooms to a plate. Wipe out the skillet with a paper towel.

In a small bowl, whisk the eggs and salt together until fluffy.

In the same skillet, melt the butter over medium-high heat, swirling to cover the bottom. Add the eggs and reduce the heat to low. As the egg cooks, lift the edges to allow the runny egg to flow underneath until the eggs are nearly set. Sprinkle 2 tablespoons of cheese over the eggs. Scatter the ham, bacon, mushrooms, tomatoes, avocado, bell pepper, yellow onion, and green onion over half of the omelet, then fold the other half over the filling. Sprinkle the top of the omelet with the remaining 1 tablespoon of cheese and the chives. Serve immediately.

4 button mushrooms, sliced
2 large eggs
Pinch salt
½ tablespoon unsalted butter
3 tablespoons shredded mozzarella cheese, divided
¼ cup diced ham
1 bacon strip, cooked and chopped
5 cherry tomatoes, halved
¼ avocado, chopped
1 tablespoon diced bell pepper
1 teaspoon diced yellow onion
1 teaspoon minced green onion
1 teaspoon minced fresh chives

Creamy Tomato Chicken Stew ⓟ ⓜ

Per serving: Calories: 334 Fat: 20g Net Carb: 10g (12%) Protein: 27g
Makes 8 servings | Prep time: 20 minutes | Cook time: 30 minutes

2 tablespoons coconut flour
1 teaspoon paprika
1 teaspoon dried oregano
1 teaspoon salt, plus more
to taste
¼ teaspoon black pepper,
plus more to taste
4 boneless, skinless
chicken breasts, halved
horizontally to make
8 cutlets
2 tablespoons unsalted
butter, divided
2 tablespoons olive oil,
divided
1 tablespoon minced garlic
1 yellow onion, halved and
sliced
8 ounces white mushrooms,
sliced
3 tablespoons tomato paste
1 (28-ounce) can crushed
tomatoes
4 cups bone broth
1 teaspoon salt
1 cup heavy cream
Fresh basil leaves, for
garnish

In a shallow bowl, combine the coconut flour, paprika, oregano, salt, and pepper. Dredge the chicken cutlets in the flour and spice mixture.

Melt 1 tablespoon of butter in 1 tablespoon of olive oil in a soup pot over medium-high heat. Add half of the chicken and brown on both sides, about 10 minutes. Transfer to a plate. Repeat with the remaining butter, olive oil, and chicken. Cut the chicken into bite-size pieces.

Reduce the heat to medium. Add the garlic and cook until fragrant, about 2 minutes. Add the onion and mushrooms and cook until soft, about 3 minutes. Add the tomato paste, crushed tomatoes, broth, and salt and bring the mixture to a simmer. Return the chicken to the pot, cover, and cook until the chicken is cooked through, about 20 minutes. Stir in the cream. Season with additional salt and pepper and garnish with fresh basil.

Tip: For a set-it-and-forget-it version of this stew, use your Instant Pot. Use the Sauté setting to brown the chicken, then remove it and cut into bite-size pieces. Return the chicken to the pot and add all the remaining ingredients except the cream. Cover and pressure-cook on high for 8 minutes, then allow for a 10-minute natural release of pressure. Remove the lid and stir in the cream.

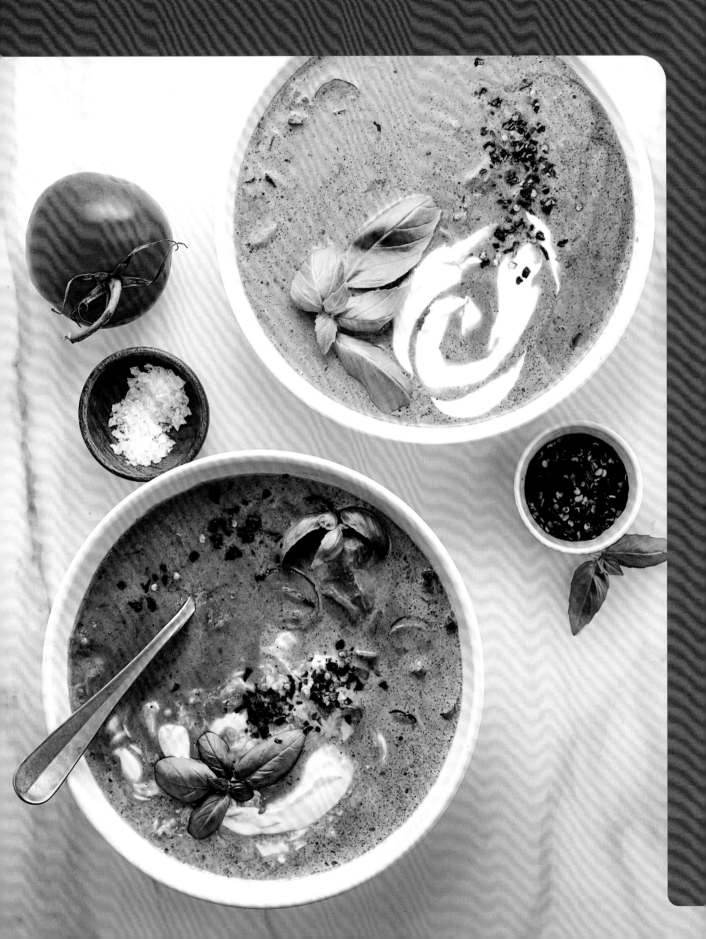

Coconut Curry Soup with Tofu Ⓟ Ⓜ

Per serving: Calories: 263 Fat: 20g Net Carb: 8g (12%) Protein: 14g
Makes 6 servings | **Prep time: 15 minutes** | **Cook time: 30 minutes**

1 tablespoon coconut oil
2 tablespoons grated fresh
  ginger
1 tablespoon minced
  lemongrass or lemongrass
  paste
1 shallot, thinly sliced
1 cup sliced red bell pepper
3 tablespoons red curry paste
4 cups bone broth
2 tablespoons coconut
  aminos or fish sauce
1 tablespoon granular
  Swerve (optional)
1 cup heavy cream
1 (14-ounce) package firm
  tofu, drained and cubed
2 tablespoons lime juice, plus
  lime wedges for serving
1 teaspoon salt
¼ teaspoon ground white
  pepper
Chopped fresh cilantro, for
  garnish
Minced red chile, for garnish
  (optional)

Heat the coconut oil in a soup pot over medium-high heat. Add the ginger, lemongrass, shallot, bell pepper, and curry paste. Sauté for 3 minutes, stirring often, until soft. Stir in the broth, coconut aminos, and Swerve (if using) and simmer for 15 minutes. Stir in the cream and tofu and simmer for 8 minutes. Stir in the lime juice, salt, and white pepper. Serve warm, garnished with cilantro and minced red chile if desired, with lime wedges for squeezing.

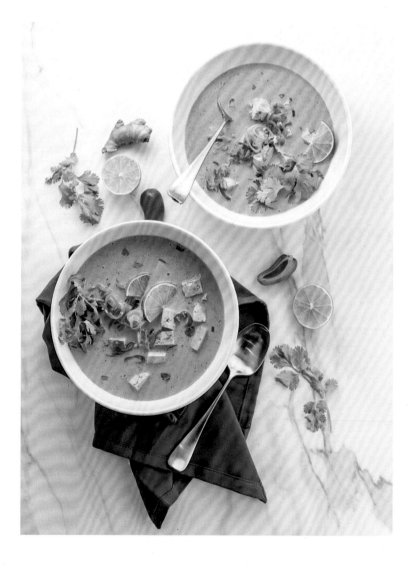

Savory Sauerkraut Soup ⓟ Ⓜ

Per serving: Calories: 304 Fat: 14g Net Carb: 11g (14%) Protein: 28g
Makes 6 servings | Prep time: 20 minutes | Cook time: 30 minutes

Heat a soup pot over medium-high heat. Add the bacon and cook until browned and crispy, about 6 minutes. Using a slotted spoon, transfer the bacon to a paper towel–lined plate, leaving the bacon drippings in the pot. When cool enough to handle, crumble the bacon.

Add the celery, garlic, and onion to the pot and sauté until soft, about 3 minutes. Add the tomato paste, paprika, Swerve, seasoning blend, marjoram, jicama, bell pepper, quinoa, and bone broth and stir. Bring to a boil for 10 minutes, then reduce to a simmer. Add the sauerkraut, salt, pepper, and about three-quarters of the bacon. Simmer for 10 minutes. Serve warm, topped with the remaining bacon, sour cream, and parsley if desired.

8 ounces bacon
2 celery ribs, diced
1 tablespoon minced garlic
1 yellow onion, diced
2 tablespoons tomato paste
1 tablespoon paprika
1 teaspoon granular Swerve
1 teaspoon salt-free Dash seasoning blend
1 teaspoon dried marjoram
½ cup cubed jicama (¼-inch cubes)
1 red bell pepper, seeded and diced
¼ cup quinoa
8 cups bone broth
3 cups sauerkraut, drained and triple rinsed
½ teaspoon salt
¼ teaspoon black pepper
Full-fat sour cream, for serving (optional)
Chopped fresh parsley, for garnish (optional)

Tip: Want to reduce the carbs in this dish to 10%? Simply omit the quinoa.

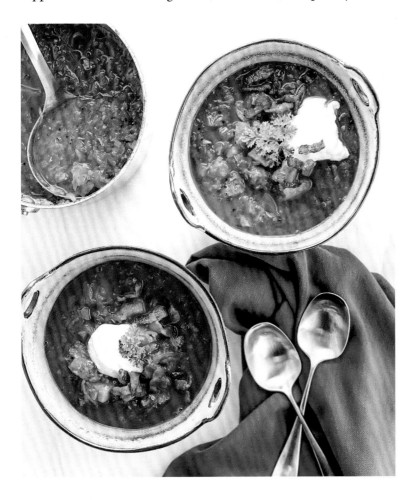

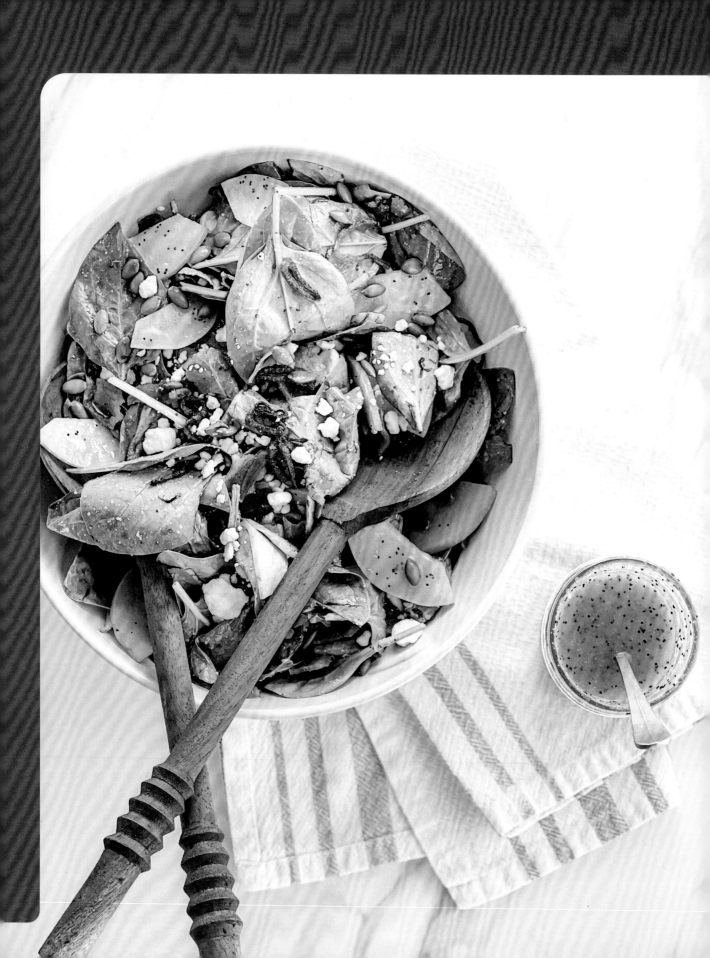

Spinach Salad with Bacon and Poppy Seed Dressing Ⓡ Ⓟ Ⓜ

Per serving: Calories: 297 Fat: 25g Net Carb: 6g (8%) Protein: 9g
Makes 4 servings | **Prep time: 15 minutes** | **Cook time: 15 minutes**

Heat a skillet over medium-high heat. Add the bacon and cook until browned and crispy, about 6 minutes. Using a slotted spoon, transfer the bacon to a paper towel–lined plate, leaving the bacon drippings in the pot. When cool enough to handle, crumble the bacon.

Reduce the heat to medium-low. Add the shallots and cook until crispy, about 20 minutes, keeping a close eye to ensure that the shallots don't burn. Transfer the shallots to the paper towel–lined plate with the bacon.

Combine the dressing ingredients in a jar with a tight-fitting lid. Secure the lid and shake the jar to combine the ingredients.

Put the spinach in a large salad bowl and toss with some of the dressing. Season with salt and pepper. Top with the sliced pear, pepitas, goat cheese, crispy shallots, and crumbled bacon.

Salad
4 slices bacon
3 shallots, thinly sliced
8 ounces baby spinach
Salt and black pepper to taste
1 Asian pear, cored and sliced
2 tablespoons roasted salted pepitas
¼ cup crumbled goat cheese

Poppy Seed Dressing
¼ cup olive oil
2 tablespoons white balsamic vinegar
2 tablespoons granulated Swerve
½ teaspoon ground mustard
½ teaspoon poppy seeds
1 teaspoon grated white onion
Pinch salt

Cobb Salad with Herb Ranch Dressing ® ℗ Ⓜ

Per serving: Calories: 454 Fat: 28g Net Carb: 7g (6%) Protein: 36g
Makes 4 servings | **Prep time: 20 minutes** | **Cook time: 10 minutes**

Salad
4 large eggs
2 heads romaine lettuce, chopped
1 cup halved cherry tomatoes
⅓ cup blue cheese crumbles
4 slices bacon, cooked and chopped
1 avocado, peeled, pitted, and sliced
2 tablespoons minced chives
2 boneless, skinless chicken breasts, cooked and sliced

Herb Ranch Dressing
¼ cup heavy cream
¼ cup sour cream
½ teaspoon minced garlic
2 teaspoons minced fresh basil
2 teaspoons minced fresh chives
½ teaspoon Italian seasoning
⅛ teaspoon ground mustard
¼ teaspoon salt
Pinch ground black pepper
¼ teaspoon apple cider vinegar

Place the eggs in a medium saucepan and pour in enough cold water to cover the eggs by about 1 inch. Bring the water to a boil over high heat. Once boiling, reduce the heat to medium and set a timer for 7 minutes. After 7 minutes, transfer the eggs to a bowl of ice water; make sure they are fully submerged. Once cool, peel and slice the eggs.

To make the dressing, in a small bowl, whisk together the heavy cream, sour cream, and minced garlic. Add the basil, chives, Italian seasoning, ground mustard, salt, and pepper and mix until fully combined. Stir in the apple cider vinegar.

Arrange the romaine lettuce on a serving platter. Top with the cherry tomatoes, blue cheese, bacon, avocado, chives, chicken, and eggs. Drizzle the dressing over the salad.

Tip: Hard-boiled eggs are an egg-cellent zero-carb food to keep on hand in the fridge. Swap out the tuna in Creamy Dill Tuna Salad for 8 chopped hard-boiled eggs and serve over lettuce leaves, wrapped in an egg tortilla (see page 136), or sandwiched in a Soft Dinner Roll (page 210).

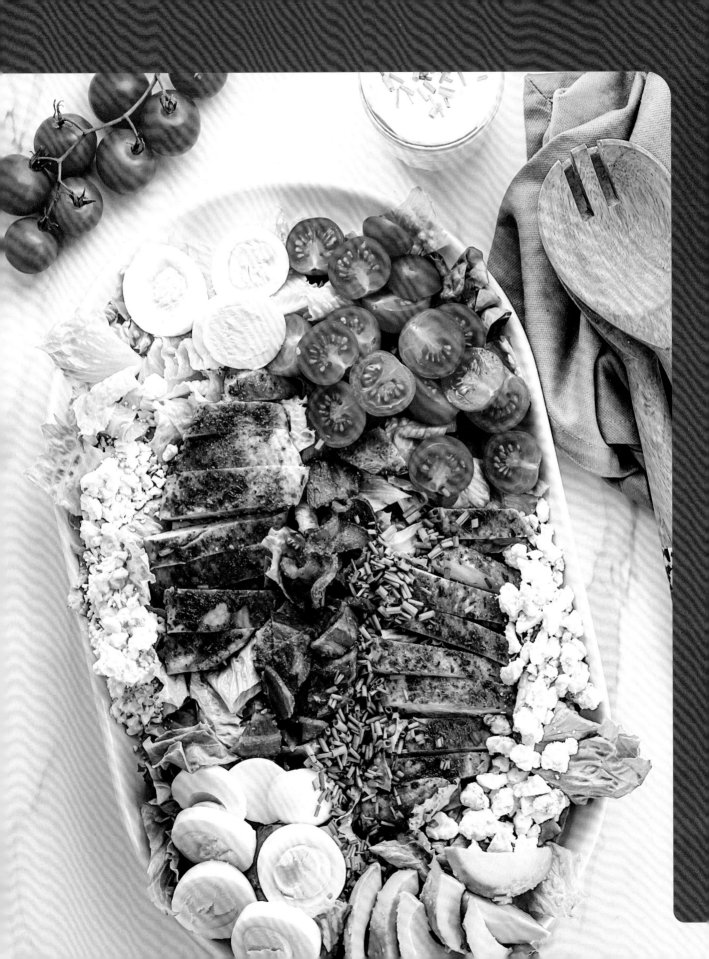

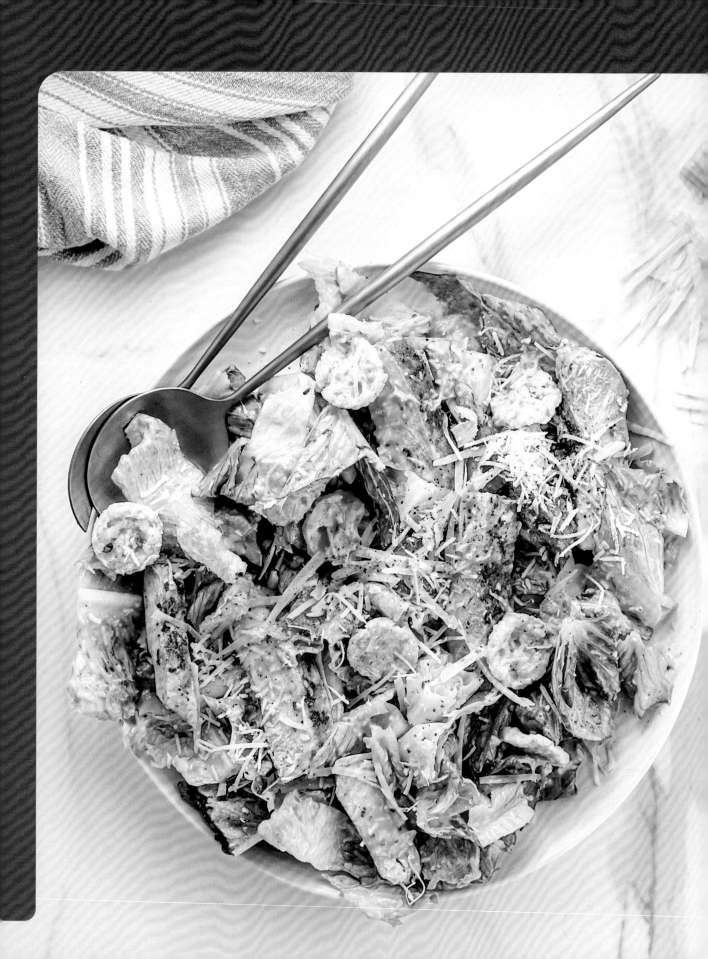

Caesar Salad with Seasoned Chicken Ⓡ Ⓟ Ⓜ

Per serving: Calories: 426 Fat: 27g Net Carb: 7g (6%) Protein: 35g
Makes 4 servings | **Prep time: 20 minutes** | **Cook time: 20 minutes**

To make the chicken, preheat the oven to 425 degrees F. Line a baking pan with parchment paper.

One at a time, place the chicken breasts between 2 sheets of parchment and pound to a ½-inch thickness.

In a small bowl, mix the Swerve, paprika, Italian seasoning, garlic powder, salt, and pepper.

Place the chicken in the prepared pan. Coat lightly with olive oil spray and sprinkle with half of the seasoning mixture. Flip the chicken and repeat by spraying with olive oil and sprinkling with the remaining seasoning mixture. Bake for 18 minutes, or until the chicken looks perfectly caramelized. Set aside to cool slightly, then slice.

To make the dressing, use a mortar and pestle to combine the anchovy fillets, garlic, and salt into a paste. In a small bowl, whisk together the egg yolk, lemon juice, and mustard. Slowly drizzle the avocado oil into the mixture while whisking, until the mixture becomes creamy. Add the Parmesan and anchovy paste. Mix well and season with salt and pepper.

In a large bowl, toss the lettuce with the dressing. Top with the grated Parmesan, Parmesan crisps, and seasoned chicken. Season with salt and pepper.

Chicken
2 boneless, skinless chicken breasts
1½ teaspoons granular Swerve
½ teaspoon paprika
½ teaspoon Italian seasoning
¼ teaspoon garlic powder
¼ teaspoon sea salt
¼ teaspoon black pepper

Caesar Dressing
2 oil-packed anchovy fillets
1 teaspoon minced garlic
½ teaspoon salt
1 large egg yolk
2 tablespoons lemon juice
1 teaspoon stone-ground mustard
¼ cup avocado oil
¼ cup grated Parmesan cheese
Salt and ground black pepper to taste

Salad
2 heads romaine lettuce, chopped
⅓ cup grated Parmesan cheese
1 (2-ounce) bag Parmesan crisps (made with cheese only, 1 gram of carbs per serving)
Salt and ground black pepper to taste

Note: Dressing contains raw egg yolk. You may wish to buy pasteurized eggs for this recipe.

Ground Beef Taco Salad Ⓡ Ⓟ Ⓜ

Per serving: Calories: 376 Fat: 25g Net Carb: 9g (9%) Protein: 27g

Makes 4 servings | **Prep time: 10 minutes** | **Cook time: 15 minutes**

1 tablespoon olive oil

1 teaspoon minced garlic

1 pound 90% lean ground beef

2 tablespoons taco seasoning

¼ cup water

1 head romaine lettuce, chopped

1 cup cherry tomatoes, halved

2 tablespoons guacamole

½ cup chopped green onion

¼ cup chopped fresh cilantro

1 cup thinly sliced jicama

1 (2.25-ounce) can sliced black olives, drained

½ cup shredded cheddar cheese

Sour cream, for garnish (optional)

Tajín seasoning, for garnish

Heat the oil in a large skillet over medium-high heat. Add the garlic and sauté until the garlic is fragrant and golden, about 2 minutes. Add the ground beef and cook, breaking it up with a wooden spoon, until no longer pink, about 8 minutes. Drain off any excess grease and liquid. Return the skillet to medium heat and add the taco seasoning and water to the ground beef. Stir to fully combine and bring to a simmer. Once all of the liquid has been absorbed, remove the skillet from the heat and set aside.

In 4 salad bowls, evenly divide the lettuce, tomatoes, guacamole, green onion, cilantro, jicama, olives, and ground beef. Top with the shredded cheddar cheese, a dollop of sour cream (if using), and a sprinkle of Tajín.

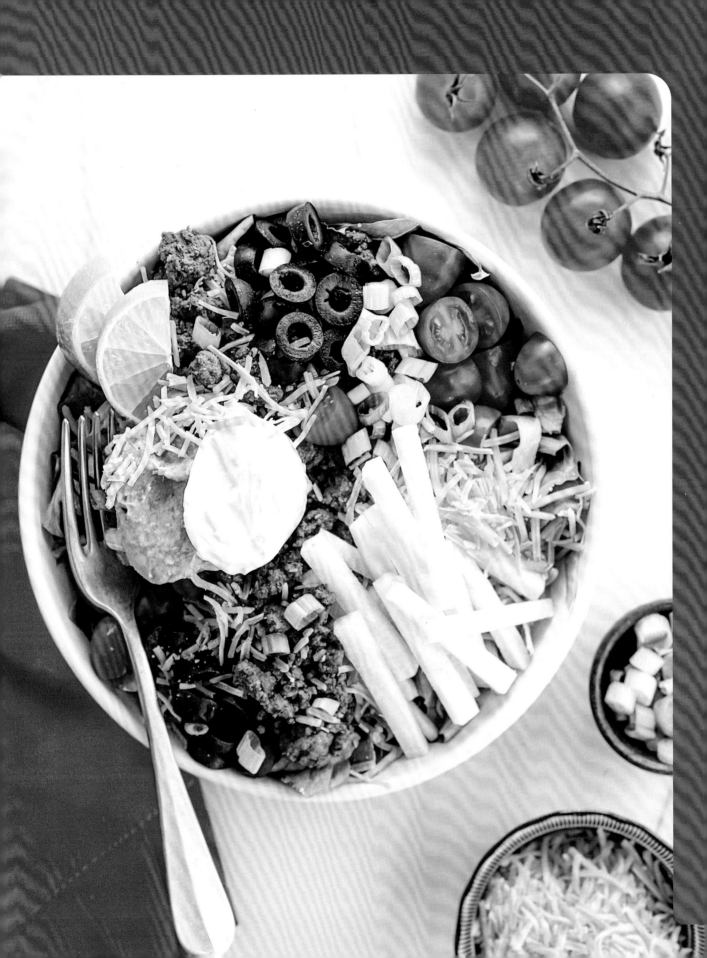

Creamy Dill Tuna Salad 🅡 🅟 🅜

Per serving: Calories: 443 Fat: 33g Net Carb: 4g (4%) Protein: 30g
Makes 4 servings | Prep time: 15 minutes

2 (6-ounce) cans albacore tuna in water

2 (6-ounce) cans albacore tuna in olive oil

⅔ cup mayonnaise

2 tablespoons yellow mustard

1 tablespoon chopped fresh dill

1 tablespoon lime juice

⅓ cup thinly sliced celery

¼ cup finely diced red onion

¼ cup diced pickle

¼ teaspoon salt

⅛ teaspoon black pepper

1 head butter lettuce

Alfalfa sprouts, for garnish (optional)

Drain the cans of tuna and flake the tuna into a large bowl. Stir in the mayo, mustard, dill, lime juice, celery, red onion, pickle, salt, and pepper. Mix until fully combined. Cover and chill until serving. Serve on top of large lettuce leaves and garnish with alfalfa sprouts if desired.

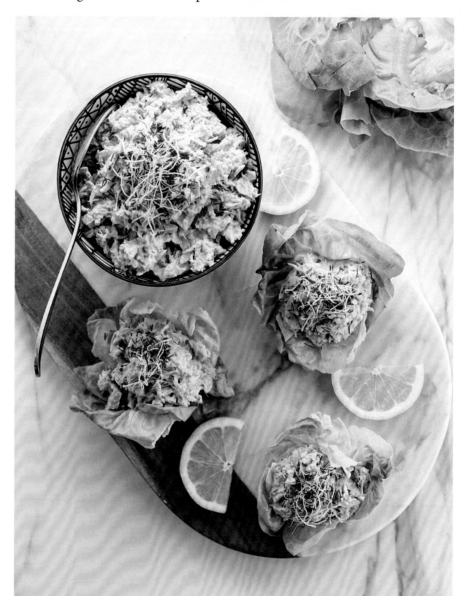

Meatzza Pizza R P M

Per serving: Calories: 432 Fat: 26g Net Carb: 4g (4%) Protein: 46g
Makes 4 servings | **Prep time: 10 minutes** | **Bake time: 30 minutes**

Preheat the oven to 400 degrees F. Line a rimmed baking sheet with parchment paper.

Combine all of the crust ingredients in a food processor and process until the chicken is fully ground and the ingredients are fully combined. Transfer the chicken mixture to the prepared baking sheet and spread it into your desired pizza shape. Bake for 20 minutes. Remove the sheet from the oven and increase the oven temperature to 500 degrees F.

Spread the sauce all over the crust, then top with the mozzarella cheese, basil, and salt. Bake for 5–8 minutes, until the cheese has melted. Serve immediately.

Crust

1 pound boneless, skinless chicken thighs
2 large eggs
½ cup shredded mozzarella cheese
¼ cup grated Parmesan cheese
1 teaspoon Italian seasoning
½ teaspoon salt

Toppings

¼ cup pizza sauce
7 ounces fresh mozzarella, sliced or chopped
8 fresh basil leaves, thinly sliced
Pinch salt

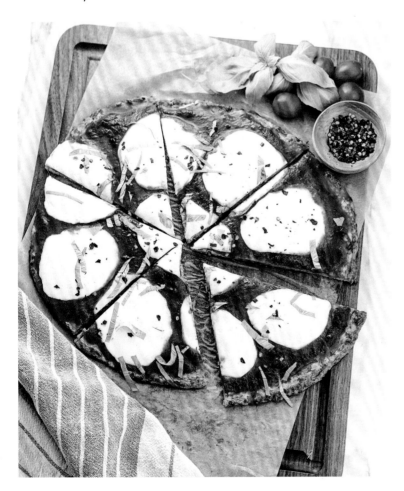

Bruschetta Skillet Chicken ⓡ ⓟ ⓜ

Per serving: Calories: 429 Fat: 25g Net Carb: 9g (8%) Protein: 40g
Makes 4 servings | **Prep time: 20 minutes** | **Cook time: 25 minutes**

Bruschetta
2 tablespoons olive oil
4 Roma tomatoes, diced
2 tablespoons finely chopped
    red onion
¼ cup thinly sliced fresh basil
½ teaspoon minced garlic
1 tablespoon balsamic
    vinegar
¼ teaspoon salt
Pinch black pepper

Spice Blend
½ cup almond flour
1 teaspoon Italian seasoning
½ teaspoon salt
⅛ teaspoon black pepper
¼ teaspoon garlic powder

Chicken
Salt and black pepper to taste
4 boneless, skinless chicken
    breasts
2 tablespoons olive oil
½ cup shaved Parmesan
    cheese
1 tablespoon balsamic
    vinegar glaze

Combine the bruschetta ingredients in a medium bowl and set aside.

Combine the spice blend ingredients in a wide, shallow bowl. Salt and pepper the chicken breasts. One at a time, place the chicken breasts between 2 sheets of parchment and pound to a ½-inch thickness. Dredge the chicken breasts in the spice blend.

Heat the oil in a large skillet over medium-high heat, swirling to cover the bottom. Reduce the heat to medium and add the chicken. Cook undisturbed for 2 minutes. Flip the chicken and reduce the heat to low. Cover and cook undisturbed for 10 minutes. Turn off the heat, but wait an additional 10 minutes before removing the lid. Check that the chicken is fully cooked; there should be no pink and a thermometer should register at least 165 degrees F.

Top the chicken breasts with equal portions of the bruschetta and shaved Parmesan cheese. Drizzle with the balsamic glaze.

Tip: If you love the flavors of tomato, basil, and balsamic vinegar as much as I do, then why not make Bruschetta Meatzza Pizza? Use the ultra-low-carb crust found on page 153, and top with this bruschetta and a drizzle of balsamic glaze.

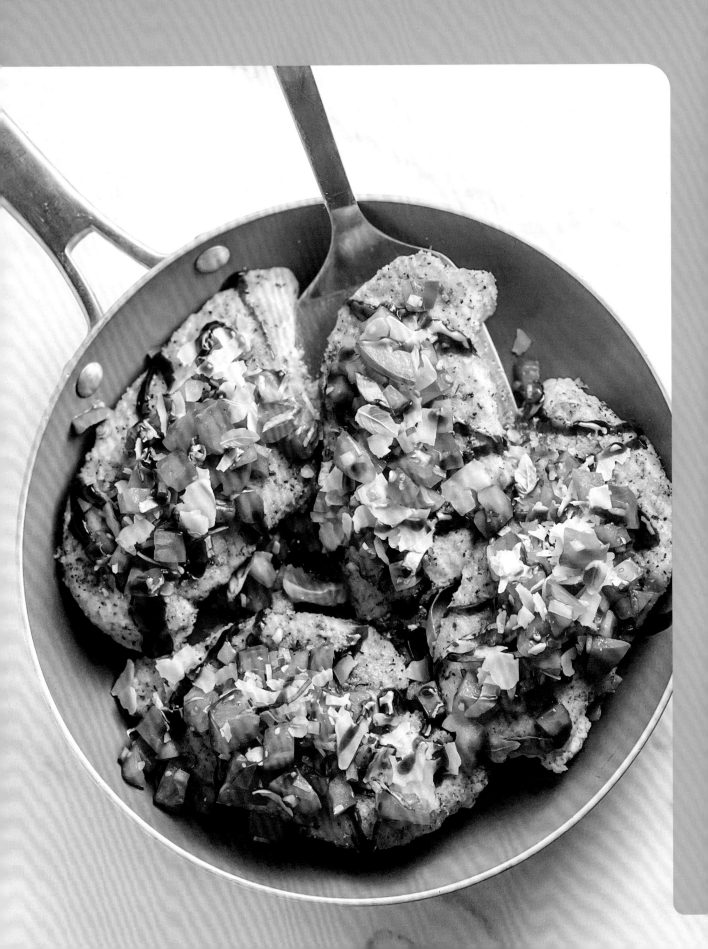

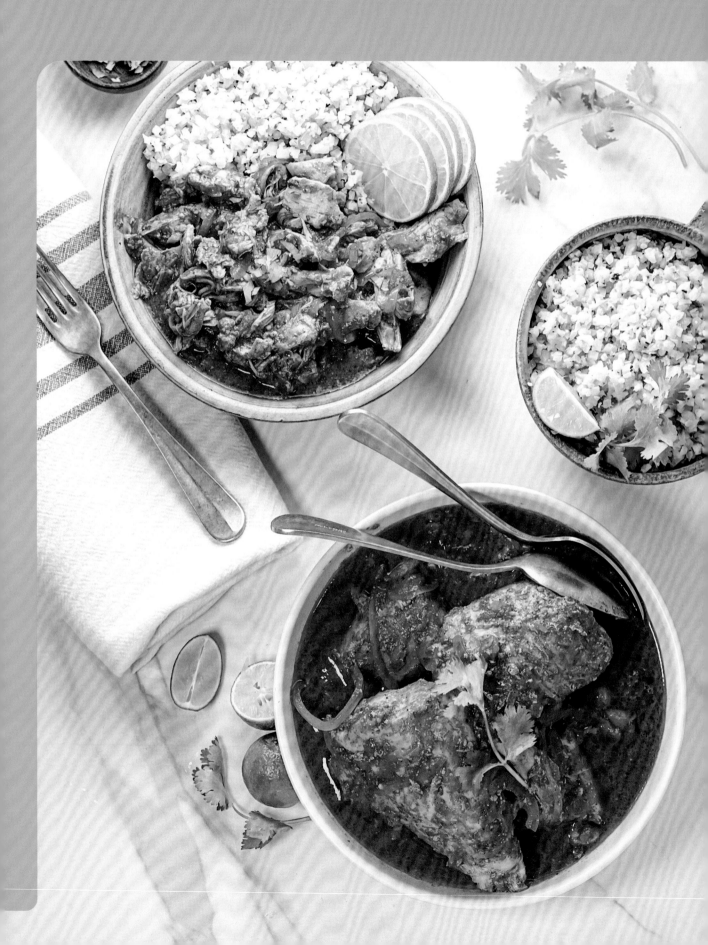

Spiced Butter Chicken Ⓡ Ⓟ Ⓜ

Per serving: Calories: 490 Fat: 29g Net Carb: 8g (6%) Protein: 50g

Makes 6 servings | Prep time: 10 minutes, plus 1 hour marinating time | Cook time: 2½–4 hours

In a medium bowl, combine the yogurt, garlic, garam masala, ginger, chili powder, and salt and mix well. Transfer the marinade to a large zip-top plastic bag and add the chicken thighs. Seal the bag and squish the chicken around until fully coated with the marinade. Refrigerate for at least 1 hour or up to overnight.

Melt the butter in a medium skillet over medium-high heat. Add the garlic and sauté until golden and fragrant, about 2 minutes. Add the onion and sauté until soft, about 3 minutes. Transfer the onion mixture to a slow cooker and top with the marinated chicken. Discard any marinade that did not stick to the chicken.

In a medium bowl, combine the tomato sauce, cream, garam masala, ginger, chili powder, and salt. Pour the sauce over the chicken. Cover and cook on low for 4 hours or on high for 2½ hours. If you like, shred the chicken before serving. Stir in the lime zest and garnish with fresh cilantro if desired.

Chicken
1 cup plain full-fat Greek yogurt
1 tablespoon chopped garlic
1 tablespoon garam masala
1 teaspoon grated fresh ginger
1 teaspoon chili powder
1 teaspoon salt
2½ pounds boneless, skinless chicken thighs

Sauce
4 tablespoons (½ stick) unsalted butter
1 tablespoon minced garlic
1 yellow onion, thinly sliced
1 (15-ounce) can tomato sauce
⅓ cup heavy cream
1 tablespoon garam masala
1 teaspoon grated fresh ginger
1 teaspoon chili powder
1 teaspoon salt
1 teaspoon grated lime zest (optional)
Fresh cilantro, for garnish (optional)

Tip: Don't want to use a slow cooker? No problem! Simply brown the marinated chicken in avocado oil in the skillet, then remove and cook the onion and garlic as directed. Once the onion is soft, mix in the remaining ingredients. Simmer for 10 minutes. Return the seared chicken to the skillet and continue to simmer for another 10 minutes, or until cooked through. Serve with cauliflower rice.

Creamy Sun-Dried Tomato Chicken ® ® Ⓜ

Per serving: Calories: 416 Fat: 23g Net Carb: 11g (10%) Protein: 38g
Makes 6 servings | **Prep time: 15 minutes** | **Cook time: 35 minutes**

8 slices bacon
3 tablespoons coconut flour
1 teaspoon dried thyme
1 teaspoon dried rosemary
Salt and black pepper to taste
2–3 pounds boneless,
  skinless chicken thighs
1 cup diced yellow onion
1 tablespoon minced garlic
⅓ cup dry white wine
1½ cups half-and-half
½ cup grated Parmesan
  cheese
4 cups baby spinach
¼ cup sun-dried tomatoes,
  packed in oil, chopped
Red pepper flakes, for
  garnish

Heat a large skillet over medium-high heat. Add the bacon and cook until crispy, about 6 minutes. Using a slotted spoon, transfer the bacon to a paper towel–lined plate. Pour off all but 2 tablespoons of bacon grease in the pan. When cool enough to handle, crumble the bacon.

In a shallow bowl, whisk together the coconut flour, thyme, and rosemary. Salt and pepper each side of the chicken thighs, then dredge in the coconut flour mixture.

Return the skillet to medium-high heat. In the bacon grease, cook the chicken thighs until cooked through, about 8 minutes per side. Transfer the chicken to a plate.

Return the skillet to medium-high heat. Add the onion, garlic, and ½ teaspoon salt and sauté until soft, about 3 minutes. Deglaze with the wine, scraping up any bits stuck to the bottom of the skillet.

Reduce the heat to low and add the half-and-half. Bring to a low simmer. Stir in the Parmesan cheese until melted. Add the spinach and sun-dried tomatoes. Stir in the chicken and bacon. Simmer for 5 minutes. Garnish with red pepper flakes.

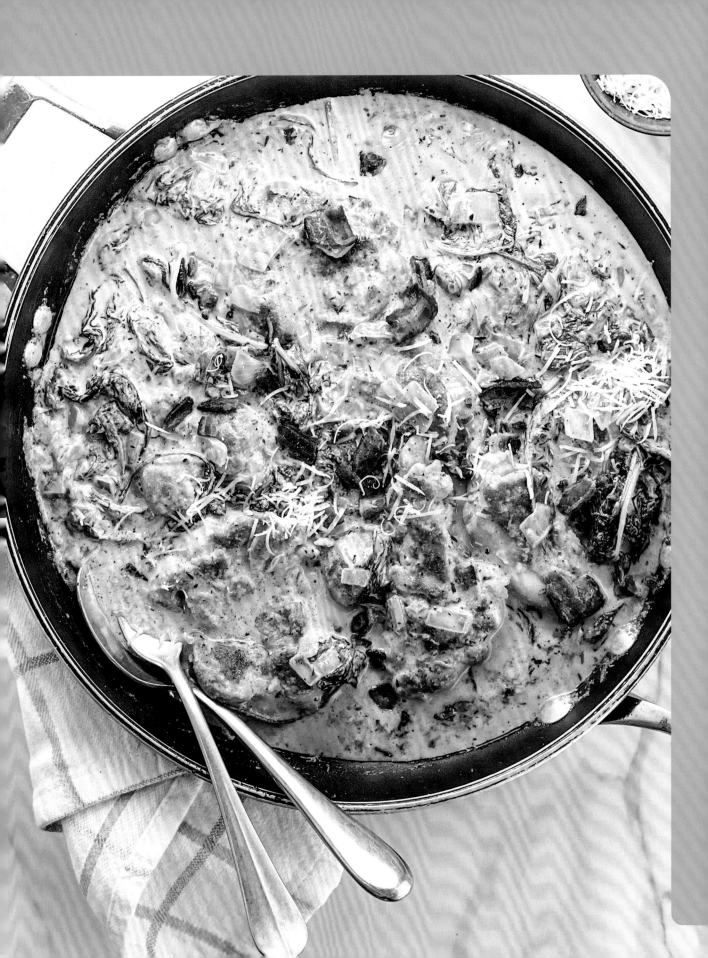

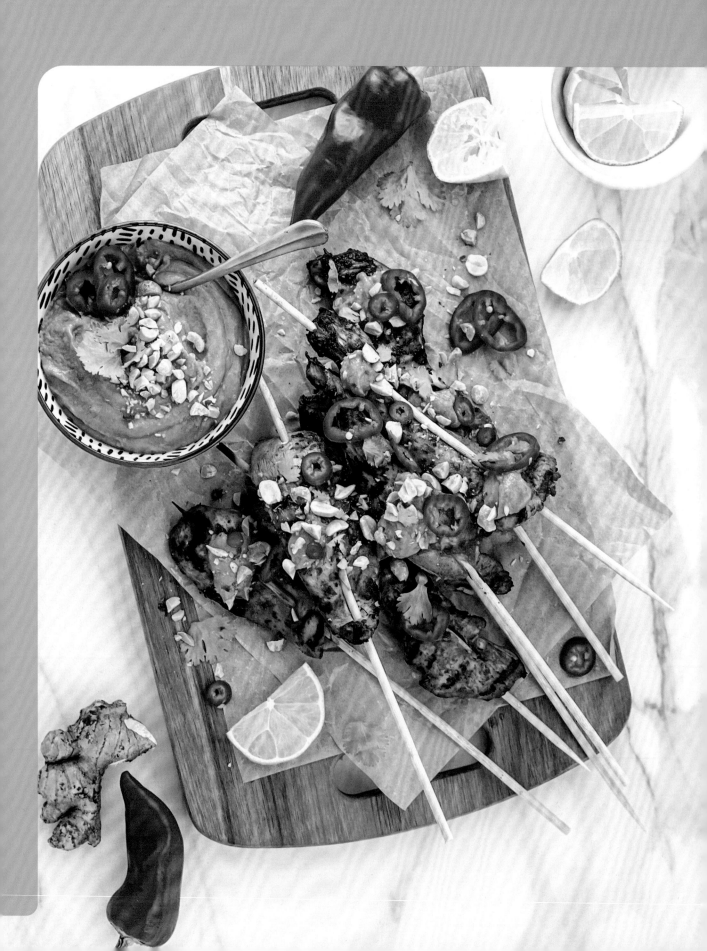

Grilled Chicken Satay with Peanut Sauce Ⓟ Ⓜ

Per serving: Calories: 307 Fat: 19g Net Carb: 9g (11%) Protein: 25g
Makes 4 servings | **Prep time: 15 minutes, plus 2 hours marinating time** | **Cook time: 15 minutes**

In a small bowl, combine the coconut milk, coconut aminos, garlic, curry powder, turmeric, ginger, granular Swerve, and fish sauce and mix well. Transfer the marinade to a large zip-top plastic bag and add the chicken strips. Seal the bag and squish the chicken around until fully coated with the marinade. Refrigerate for at least 2 hours or up to overnight.

About 30 minutes before you're ready to cook, soak wooden skewers in water (or use metal skewers).

In a small bowl, combine all of the peanut sauce ingredients and whisk until smooth. Set aside until ready to serve.

Heat an outdoor grill or stovetop grill pan over medium-high heat. Thread the chicken strips onto the skewers. Grill until cooked through, about 6 minutes per side. Top with the chopped peanuts, cilantro, and red chile slices and serve with the peanut sauce.

Chicken
¼ cup full-fat coconut milk
2 tablespoons coconut aminos or soy sauce
1 tablespoon minced garlic
2 teaspoons yellow curry powder
2 teaspoons ground turmeric
1 teaspoon grated fresh ginger
1 teaspoon granular Swerve
1 teaspoon fish sauce
2 pounds boneless, skinless chicken breasts, cut into 1-inch strips

Peanut Sauce
⅓ cup creamy peanut butter
1 tablespoon coconut aminos or soy sauce
1 tablespoon lime juice
¼ teaspoon salt
2 teaspoons brown Swerve
1 tablespoon chili garlic sauce
1 teaspoon grated fresh ginger
3 tablespoons full-fat coconut milk

Toppings
1 tablespoon chopped peanuts
1 tablespoon chopped fresh cilantro
1 tablespoon thinly sliced red chiles

Chicken Alfredo Spaghetti Bake Ⓟ Ⓜ

Per serving: Calories: 483 Fat: 35g Net Carb: 16g (13%) Protein: 25g
Makes 6 servings | **Prep time: 15 minutes** | **Cook time: 45 minutes**

Spaghetti Bake

2 large eggs
⅓ cup sour cream
1 teaspoon salt
1 teaspoon Italian seasoning
¼ teaspoon black pepper
½ teaspoon garlic powder
4 cups cooked spaghetti squash (see box)
4 cups shredded cooked chicken
1 cup shredded mozzarella cheese
¼ cup grated Parmesan cheese (must be fresh!)

Alfredo Sauce

4 tablespoons (½ stick) unsalted butter
1 cup heavy cream
1 teaspoon minced garlic
1½ cups grated Parmesan cheese (must be fresh!)
¼ cup minced fresh parsley

Preheat the oven to 375 degrees F. Coat a 9 × 13-inch baking pan with cooking spray.

In a large bowl, whisk together the eggs, sour cream, salt, Italian seasoning, black pepper, and garlic powder. Add the spaghetti squash strands and shredded chicken and mix well. Stir in the mozzarella and Parmesan cheeses. Press the mixture into the prepared baking pan.

Melt the butter in a small skillet over medium-low heat. Add the cream and bring to a simmer; simmer for 5 minutes. Add the garlic and Parmesan, whisking until melted. Pour two-thirds of the sauce over the prepared casserole, reserving the rest of the sauce for serving.

Bake for 35 minutes, or until bubbly and golden. Garnish with the parsley and serve with the reserved sauce.

Cooking Spaghetti Squash: Preheat the oven to 450 degrees F. Line a rimmed baking sheet with parchment paper. Cut 2 spaghetti squash in half lengthwise. Scoop out and discard the seeds. Season the cut sides of the squash halves with salt and pepper and rub with coconut oil or avocado oil. Place the squash halves, cut side down, on the prepared baking sheet. Bake for 30–40 minutes until tender, then let cool. Scoop the cooked spaghetti squash into a colander and press down with a paper towel to drain into the sink.

Tip: To bring the carbs down to 10%, reduce the spaghetti squash to 3 cups.

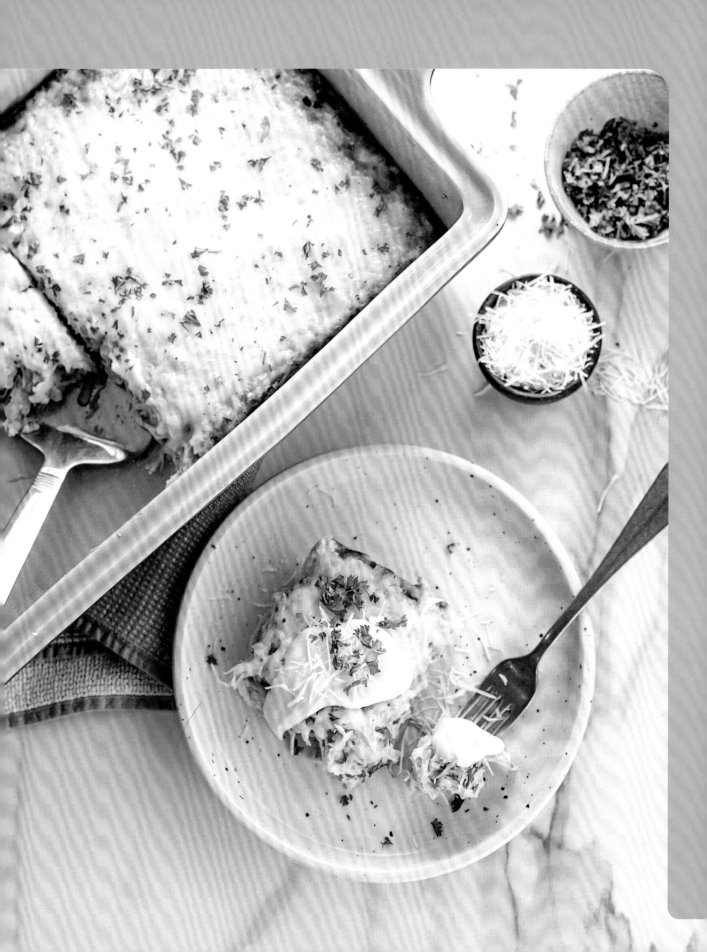

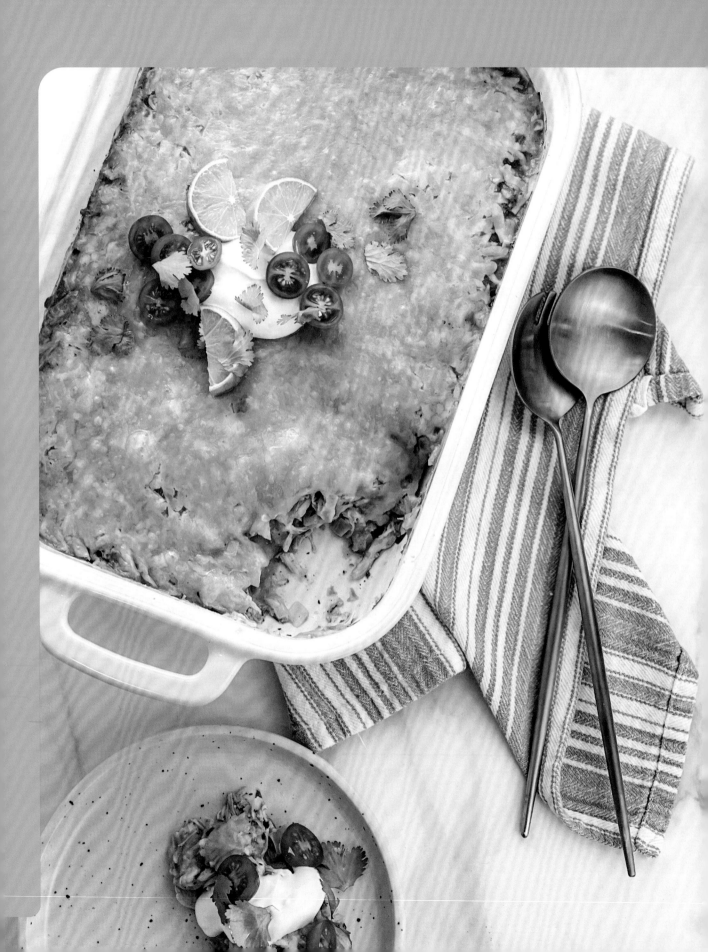

Easy Chicken Enchilada Casserole 🅡 🅟 🅜

Per serving: Calories: 506 Fat: 28g Net Carb: 9g (7%) Protein: 52g
Makes 6 servings | **Prep time: 15 minutes** | **Cook time: 35 minutes**

Preheat the oven to 350 degrees F.

Heat the oil in a medium skillet over medium-high heat. Add the garlic and cook until fragrant, about 2 minutes. Add the onion and cook until soft, about 3 minutes. Stir in the chiles. Stir in the cream cheese until melted, then remove the pan from the heat.

Put the shredded chicken in a large bowl. Stir in the cilantro, fajita seasoning, salt, and pepper. Add the cream cheese mixture and mix until fully combined.

Spread ¼ cup of enchilada sauce in the bottom of a 9 × 13-inch baking pan. Add the chicken mixture. Top with the remaining sauce and sprinkle with the shredded cheese. Bake for 20–25 minutes, until the cheese is melted. Serve topped with sour cream, cherry tomatoes, more cilantro, and lime wedges, if desired.

1 tablespoon olive oil

1 teaspoon minced garlic

1 yellow onion, diced

1 (4-ounce) can diced mild green chiles, drained

4 ounces cream cheese

8 cups shredded cooked chicken (about 2 pounds)

¼ cup minced fresh cilantro, plus more for garnish (optional)

1 tablespoon fajita seasoning

1 teaspoon salt

½ teaspoon black pepper

1 (14-ounce) can enchilada sauce

1 cup shredded Mexican-style four-cheese blend

Sour cream, for garnish (optional)

Cherry tomatoes, chopped, for garnish (optional)

Lime wedges, for garnish (optional)

Tip: Feeling like adding some tortillas to this enchilada casserole? Make 6 of the egg tortillas on page 136. After spreading ¼ cup of the sauce in the baking pan, roll the chicken filling inside the tortillas. Place in the pan, seam side down, and top with the remaining enchilada sauce and cheese. Bake as directed.

Cinnamon Spiced Chicken Curry Ⓡ Ⓟ Ⓜ

Per serving: Calories: 380 Fat: 26g Net Carb: 7g (8%) Protein: 31g
Makes 6 servings | **Prep time: 20 minutes** | **Cook time: 40 minutes**

2 tablespoons coconut oil

1 tablespoon minced garlic

1 red onion, sliced

1 tablespoon minced fresh
    ginger

2 tablespoons curry powder

1 tablespoon paprika

½ teaspoon cayenne pepper

2 cups thinly sliced dinosaur
    kale

3 vine-ripened tomatoes,
    chopped

1 teaspoon brown Swerve

1 cinnamon stick

2 bay leaves

Salt and black pepper to taste

2–3 pounds bone-in chicken
    thighs, skin removed

2 teaspoons apple cider
    vinegar

1 (13.5-ounce) can full-fat
    coconut milk

Chopped fresh cilantro, for
    garnish (optional)

Heat the coconut oil in a large Dutch oven over medium-high heat. Add the garlic and sauté until fragrant, about 2 minutes. Add the onion, ginger, curry powder, paprika, and cayenne and sauté until aromatic, about 2 minutes. Stir in the kale, tomatoes, Swerve, cinnamon stick, bay leaves, and ½ teaspoon salt and cook for 10 minutes.

Season the chicken thighs with salt and black pepper on both sides. Add to the pot, along with the vinegar and coconut milk. Bring to a simmer. Cover, reduce the heat to medium-low, and cook for 20 minutes. Remove the bay leaves and cinnamon stick. Garnish with cilantro (if using) and serve.

Tip: This recipe is perfect for the slow cooker. Once the sauce is made, instead of adding the chicken thighs to the pot, place the chicken thighs in a slow cooker and cover with the sauce. Cover and cook on low for 5–6 hours or on high for 3–4 hours. Serve with steamed rice or cauliflower rice.

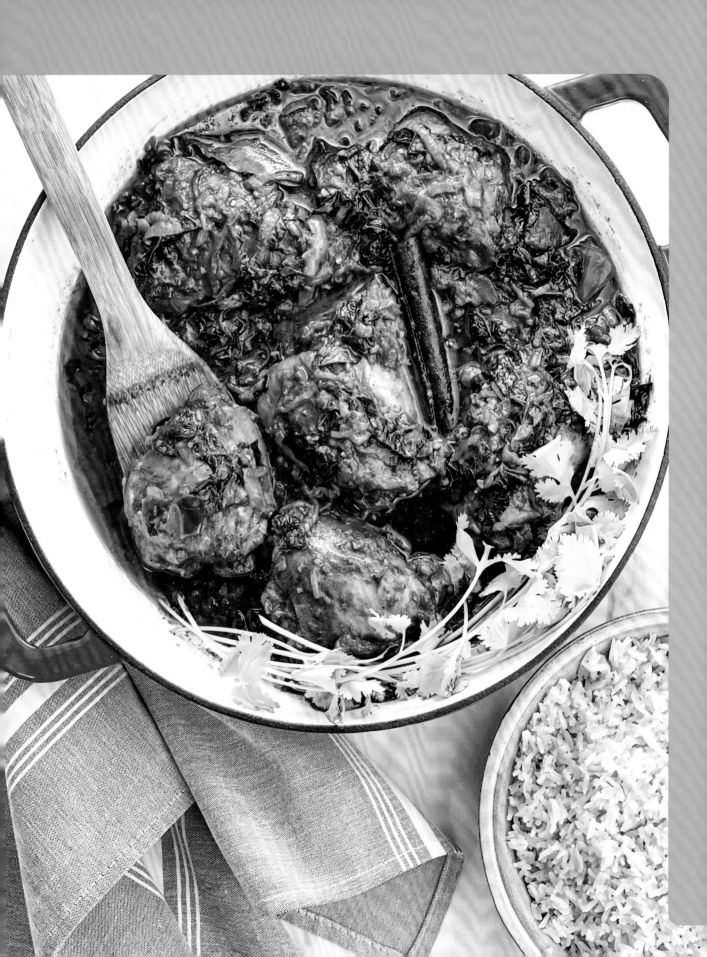

Red Wine Braised Turkey Legs ⓡ ⓟ ⓜ

Per serving: Calories: 491 Fat: 20g Net Carb: 10g (8%) Protein: 44g
Makes 4 servings | Prep time: 20 minutes | Cook time: 4 hours

2 bone-in, skin-on whole turkey legs (or 2 thighs and 2 drumsticks)

Salt and black pepper to taste

2 tablespoons olive oil

8 ounces pearl onions, peeled

2 celery ribs, roughly chopped

1 tablespoon minced garlic

4 thyme sprigs

2 rosemary sprigs

2 cups dry red wine

2 bay leaves

2 cups bone broth

1 tablespoon cornstarch or agar powder

2 tablespoons water

Tip: This recipe does well in the slow cooker. Instead of putting the skillet in the oven, transfer the contents to a slow cooker, cover, and cook on low for 6-8 hours or on high for 3-4 hours.

Preheat the oven to 275 degrees F.

Season the turkey legs generously with salt and pepper on all sides. Heat the olive oil in a large oven-safe skillet over high heat. Add the turkey legs, skin side down, and cook until deep golden brown, about 8 minutes. Flip the legs and cook until the second side is browned, about 5 minutes. Transfer the turkey to a plate.

Add the onions, celery, garlic, thyme, and rosemary to the skillet and cook, stirring frequently, until the vegetables are golden, about 8 minutes.

Add the wine, bring to a boil, and cook until reduced by half, about 5 minutes. Add the bay leaves and bone broth and bring to a boil. Return the turkey legs to the pan, placing them on top of the vegetables so that only the skin is exposed. Transfer the skillet to the oven and bake until the skin is deep mahogany, the meat is fall-apart tender, and the sauce is reduced, 3–4 hours. Every 30 minutes, spoon some of the sauce over the turkey. If the skin is turning too brown before the meat is tender, cover the pan with aluminum foil.

Transfer the turkey legs and onions to a platter; discard the herb sprigs and bay leaves. Using an immersion blender, blend the cooking juices until smooth. Transfer the blended juices to a small skillet and set over medium-low heat. In a small bowl, whisk together the cornstarch and water. Whisk the cornstarch mixture into the blended juices, then simmer until thickened. Serve the turkey with the onions and gravy.

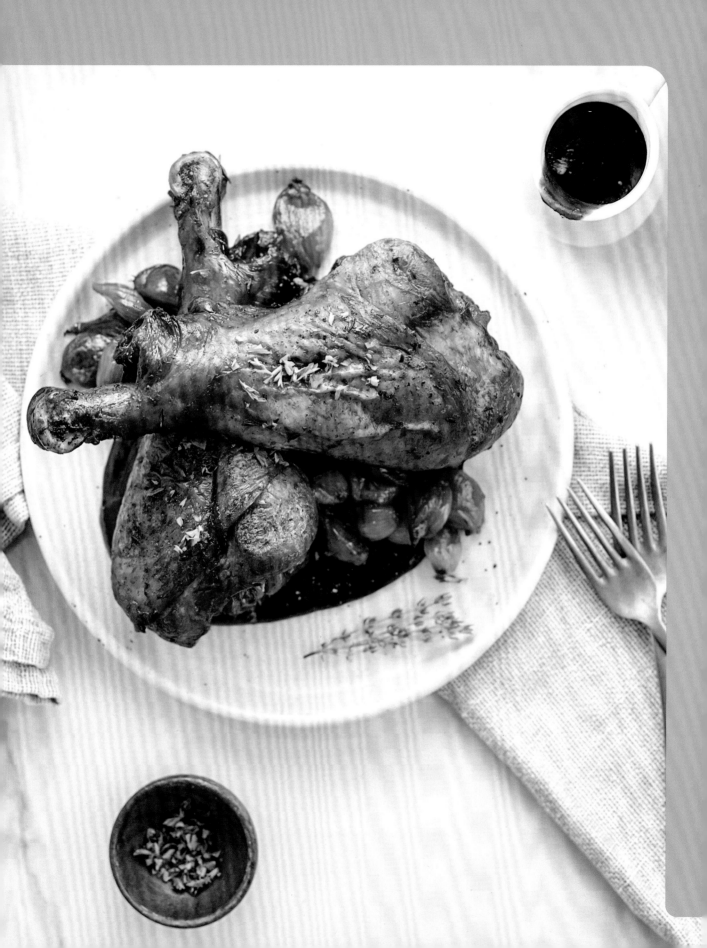

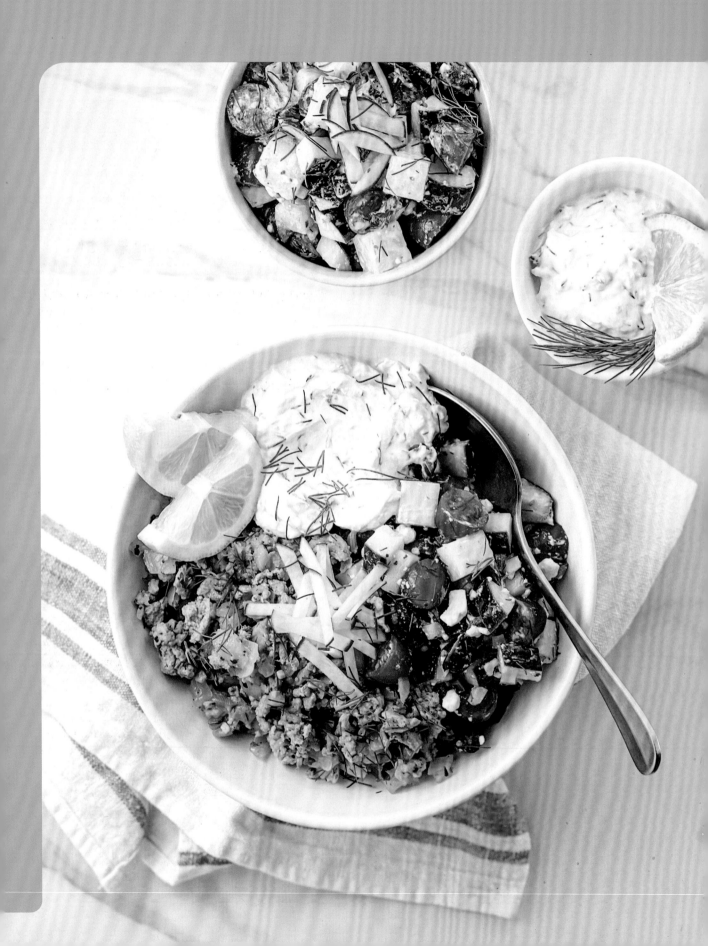

Mediterranean Turkey Bowls ® ℗ Ⓜ

Per serving: Calories: 486 Fat: 37g Net Carb: 10g (8%) Protein: 25g
Makes 4 servings | **Prep time: 20 minutes** | **Cook time: 15 minutes**

To make the turkey, heat the oil in a large skillet over medium-high heat. Add the garlic and onion and sauté until soft, about 3 minutes. Add the ground turkey and cook, breaking it up with a wooden spoon, until browned, about 8 minutes. Stir in the Italian seasoning, salt, pepper, and lemon juice.

To make the yogurt sauce, combine all the ingredients in a medium bowl and stir until fully combined.

To make the cucumber salad, in a medium bowl combine the cucumber, olives, tomatoes, feta cheese, onion, and parsley. In a small bowl, whisk together all the dressing ingredients and pour over the salad. Toss until well coated.

Divide the turkey mixture and cucumber salad evenly into 4 bowls. Add a dollop of yogurt sauce to each and garnish with the parsley, feta cheese, lemon slices, and radishes.

Turkey
2 tablespoons olive oil
1 tablespoon minced garlic
½ cup diced yellow onion
1 pound ground turkey
1 tablespoon Italian seasoning
½ teaspoon salt
¼ teaspoon black pepper
Dash lemon juice
¼ cup chopped fresh parsley
¼ cup crumbled feta cheese
1 lemon, sliced, for garnish (optional)
4 radishes, sliced, for garnish (optional)

Yogurt Sauce
⅓ cup grated cucumber, drained
½ cup plain full-fat Greek yogurt
2 teaspoons lemon juice
2 teaspoons olive oil
¼ teaspoon grated garlic
⅛ teaspoon salt
1 tablespoon minced fresh dill

Cucumber Salad
1 large cucumber, diced
¼ cup halved pitted Kalamata olives
1 cup halved cherry tomatoes
¼ cup crumbled feta cheese
¼ cup minced red onion
1 tablespoon minced fresh parsley

Dill Dressing
¼ cup olive oil
2 tablespoons red wine vinegar
1 tablespoon minced fresh dill
½ teaspoon granular Swerve
½ teaspoon minced garlic
½ teaspoon dried Italian seasoning
⅛ teaspoon salt

Meat

Favorite Lamb Larb 🅡 🅟 🅜

Per serving: Calories: 373 Fat: 25g Net Carb: 7g (8%) Protein: 40g
Makes 6 servings | Prep time: 15 minutes | Cook time: 15 minutes

⅓ cup coconut aminos or soy sauce
2 tablespoons granular Swerve
2 teaspoons fish sauce
1 teaspoon sambal oelek or other chili paste
2 tablespoons coconut oil
1 large yellow onion, finely chopped
1 green chile, seeded and minced
1 tablespoon minced garlic
2 pounds ground lamb
½ cup chopped fresh cilantro, divided
¼ teaspoon salt
2 teaspoons grated lime zest
2 tablespoons lime juice
4 green onions, chopped
1 red bell pepper, diced

In a small bowl, whisk together the coconut aminos, Swerve, fish sauce, and sambal oelek; set aside.

Heat the coconut oil in a large skillet over medium-high heat. Add the yellow onion and minced chile and cook until the onion softens, about 3 minutes. Add the garlic and cook for another minute. Add the lamb and cook, breaking it up, until no longer pink, about 8 minutes. Drain off any excess grease and liquid. Add the coconut amino mixture, ¼ cup of cilantro, and the salt. Cook, stirring often, until the pan is almost dry, about 2 minutes.

Remove the pan from the heat and add the lime zest and juice. Mix well and season to taste. Serve topped with the green onions, bell pepper, and remaining ¼ cup of cilantro.

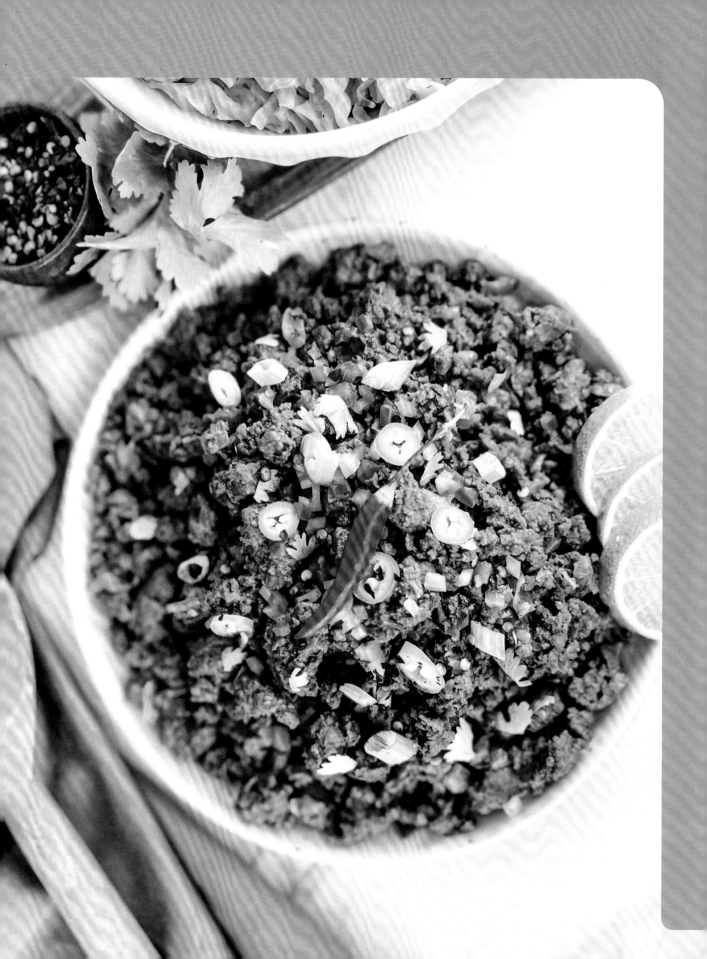

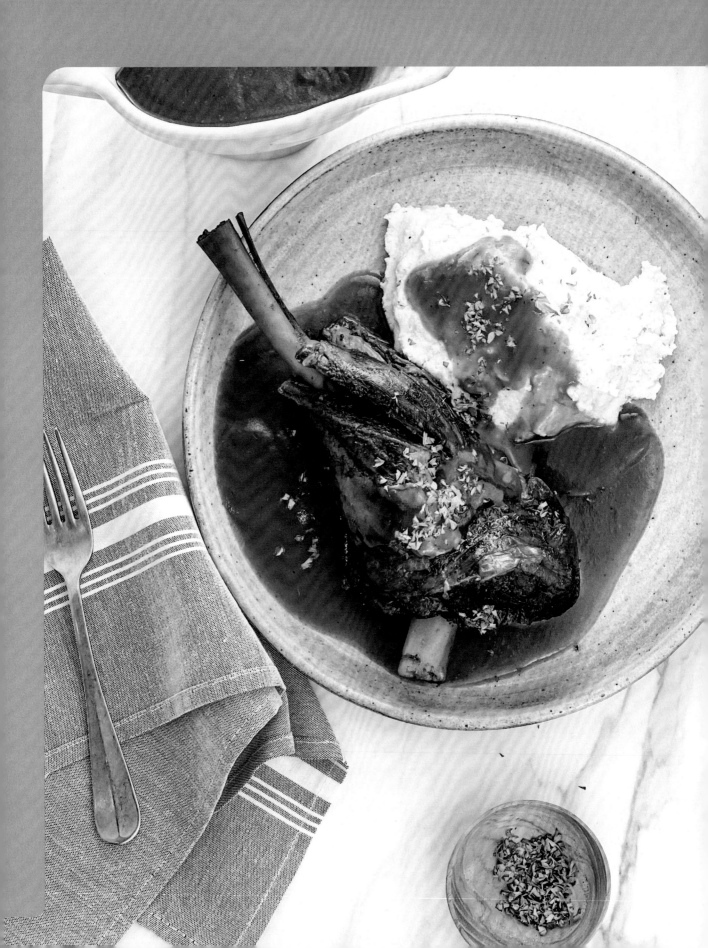

Braised Lamb Shanks with Gravy ⓡ ⓟ ⓜ

Per serving: Calories: 503 Fat: 22g Net Carb: 13g (10%) Protein: 33g
Makes 4 servings | Prep time: 20 minutes | Cook time: 8½ hours

Season the lamb shanks generously with the salt and pepper on all sides. Heat 1 tablespoon of olive oil in a large skillet over high heat. Add the lamb shanks and cook until browned on the bottom, about 8 minutes. Flip and cook until the second side is browned, about 5 minutes. Transfer to the slow cooker.

Return the skillet to medium-high heat and deglaze with 2 tablespoons of red wine. Add the remaining 1 tablespoon of olive oil, the garlic, onion, celery, and parsnip and cook until softened, about 10 minutes. Stir in the tomato paste, Worcestershire sauce, and remaining 2 cups of red wine. Simmer for 5 minutes. Pour the sauce over the lamb. Cover and cook on low for 8 hours.

Turn on the broiler. Transfer the shanks to a broiler-safe baking pan. Broil until browned, about 5 minutes.

Meanwhile, using a handheld immersion blender, blend the veggies and sauce in the slow cooker until smooth. Transfer the gravy to a skillet and heat over medium-low heat. In a small bowl, whisk together the cornstarch and water, then whisk the mixture into the blended sauce and simmer until thickened, about 5 minutes. Serve the lamb shanks with gravy and sprinkle with minced parsley.

- 4 lamb shanks (about 4 pounds total)
- 1 teaspoon salt
- ½ teaspoon black pepper
- 2 tablespoons olive oil, divided
- 2 cups plus 2 tablespoons dry red wine, divided
- 1 tablespoon minced garlic
- 1 yellow onion, cut into large pieces
- 3 celery ribs, cut into large pieces
- 1 large parsnip, peeled and cut into large pieces
- 2 tablespoons tomato paste
- 2 tablespoons Worcestershire sauce
- 1 tablespoon cornstarch or agar powder
- 2 tablespoons water
- 2 tablespoons minced parsley

Tip: You can braise these lamb shanks in the oven, if you'd prefer. Preheat the oven to 275 degrees F. After browning, transfer the lamb shanks to a plate, then return them to the skillet after cooking the vegetables. Put the skillet in the oven and bake until tender, 3–4 hours. Every 30 minutes, spoon some sauce over the shanks. If the shanks get too brown, cover the skillet. Serve with Better-Than-Mashed-Potatoes (page 214).

BBQ Pulled Pork Sliders Ⓡ Ⓟ Ⓜ

Per serving (with dinner roll): Calories: 664 Fat: 49g Net Carb: 11g (7%) Protein: 49g
Per serving (without dinner roll): Calories: 504 Fat: 37g Net Carb: 4g (3%) Protein: 34g
Makes 12 servings | **Prep time: 15 minutes** | **Cook time: 8 hours**

Pork Roast
2 tablespoons brown Swerve
2 tablespoons smoked
  paprika
1 tablespoon dried oregano
1 tablespoon ground cumin
2 teaspoons salt
1 teaspoon black pepper
1 (5-pound) pork shoulder
  roast
1 white onion, chopped
1 tablespoon minced garlic
1 cup bone broth
No-sugar-added barbecue
  sauce (optional)

Coleslaw
¼ cup mayonnaise
2 tablespoons apple cider
  vinegar
2 tablespoons granular
  Swerve
½ teaspoon celery seed
¼ teaspoon salt
Pinch white pepper
4 cups shredded cabbage or
  packaged coleslaw mix

Sliders
12 Soft Dinner Rolls (page
  210; optional)
No-sugar-added pickle chips,
  chopped (optional)
Shredded mozzarella
  (optional)

Tip: Sliders are super fun, but
you can also serve this tasty
BBQ pulled pork in a bowl
topped with the coleslaw.

In a small bowl, mix together the Swerve, smoked paprika, oregano, cumin, salt, and black pepper. Rub the spice blend all over the roast. Place the roast in a slow cooker. Top with the onion, garlic, and broth. Cover and cook on high for 8 hours.

Remove the roast from the slow cooker and shred. Season with salt and the BBQ sauce if desired.

In a large bowl, mix together the mayonnaise, vinegar, Swerve, celery seed, salt, and white pepper. Add the shredded cabbage and toss to coat.

Serve the pulled pork on the rolls, topped with coleslaw, pickles, mozzarella, and additional barbecue sauce if desired.

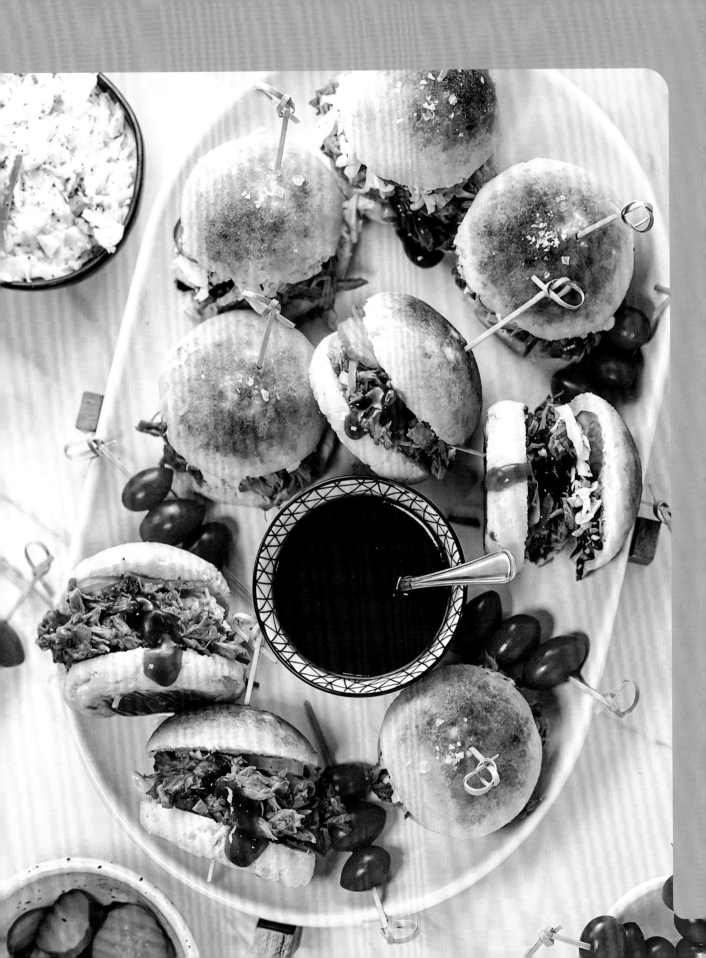

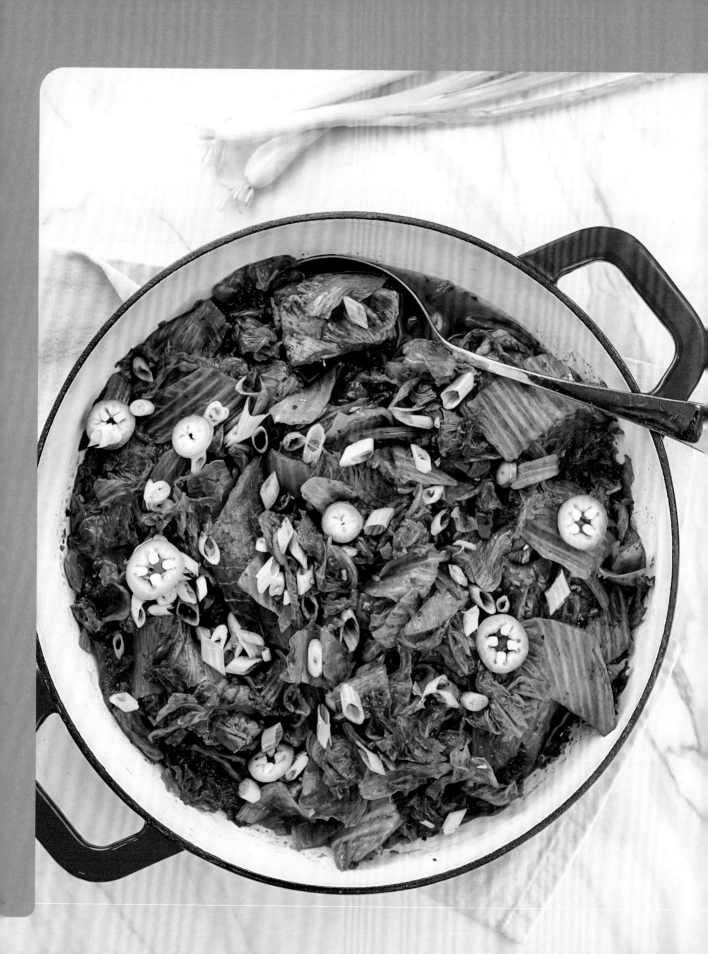

Fall-Off-the-Bone Kimchi Pork Ribs ⓡ ⓟ ⓜ

Per serving: Calories: 404 Fat: 30g Net Carb: 4g (4%) Protein: 25g
Makes 6 servings | Prep time: 30 minutes | Cook time: 2 hours

Soak the ribs in cold water for 20 minutes. Drain. Meanwhile, bring a large pot of water to a boil. Add the soybean paste and pork ribs. Boil for 8 minutes. Drain and rinse the ribs; rinse the pot.

In the pot, combine the water, dried anchovies, and ginger. Bring to a boil and boil for 15 minutes. Strain out and discard the ginger and dried anchovies; set the stock aside.

In a large bowl, combine the kimchi liquid, coconut aminos, garlic, red pepper flakes, Swerve, and sesame oil and mix well. Add the pork ribs and toss in the sauce.

Transfer 2 cups of stock to a Dutch oven and add the onion. Top with the pork ribs and kimchi. Bring to a boil, then reduce the heat to medium-low, cover, and cook for 40 minutes. Flip the kimchi pieces over, add more stock as needed, cover, and cook until the pork is tender, another 45 minutes. Top with the jalapeño and green onions.

4 pounds bone-in pork spareribs
1 tablespoon soybean paste
5 cups water
6 dried anchovies
1 (1-inch) piece fresh ginger, thinly sliced
2 tablespoons kimchi liquid
1 tablespoon coconut aminos or soy sauce
1 tablespoon minced garlic
1 teaspoon red pepper flakes
1 teaspoon granular Swerve
1 teaspoon toasted sesame oil
1 white onion, sliced
4 cups kimchi
1 jalapeño seeded and sliced
3 green onions, sliced

Pork Tenderloin with Gravy Ⓡ Ⓟ Ⓜ

Per serving: Calories: 391 Fat: 16g Net Carb: 9g (9%) Protein: 48g
Makes 4 servings | Prep time: 10 minutes | Cook time: 4 hours

Pork
1 tablespoon olive oil
2 (1¼-pound) pork
  tenderloins
1 tablespoon cornstarch or
  agar powder
2 tablespoons water

Marinade
½ cup chicken, beef, or
  vegetable broth
⅓ cup coconut aminos or soy
  sauce
3 tablespoons
  Worcestershire sauce
2 tablespoons lemon juice
1 tablespoon brown Swerve
1 tablespoon dried basil
2 teaspoons onion powder
2 teaspoons garlic powder
1 teaspoon minced garlic
½ teaspoon white pepper
¼ teaspoon cayenne pepper

Heat the oil in a large skillet over medium-high heat. Add the pork tenderloins and sear on each side until golden, about 6 minutes. Transfer the tenderloins to a slow cooker.

In a medium bowl, combine all of the marinade ingredients and mix well. Pour the marinade over the tenderloins. Cover and cook on high for 4 hours, or until the internal temperature reaches 150–160 degrees F. Transfer the braising liquid to a skillet and heat over medium-low heat. In a small bowl, whisk together the cornstarch and water, then whisk the mixture into the braising liquid. Simmer until thickened, about 5 minutes. Serve the tenderloins with the gravy.

Tip: This tenderloin is also wonderful grilled, without gravy. Marinate the tenderloin in half of the marinade for 30 minutes, reserving the other half. Preheat a grill to medium and oil the grates. Drain the pork (discard the used marinade) and grill, covered, for 15–20 minutes, turning every 5 minutes and brushing with the reserved marinade.

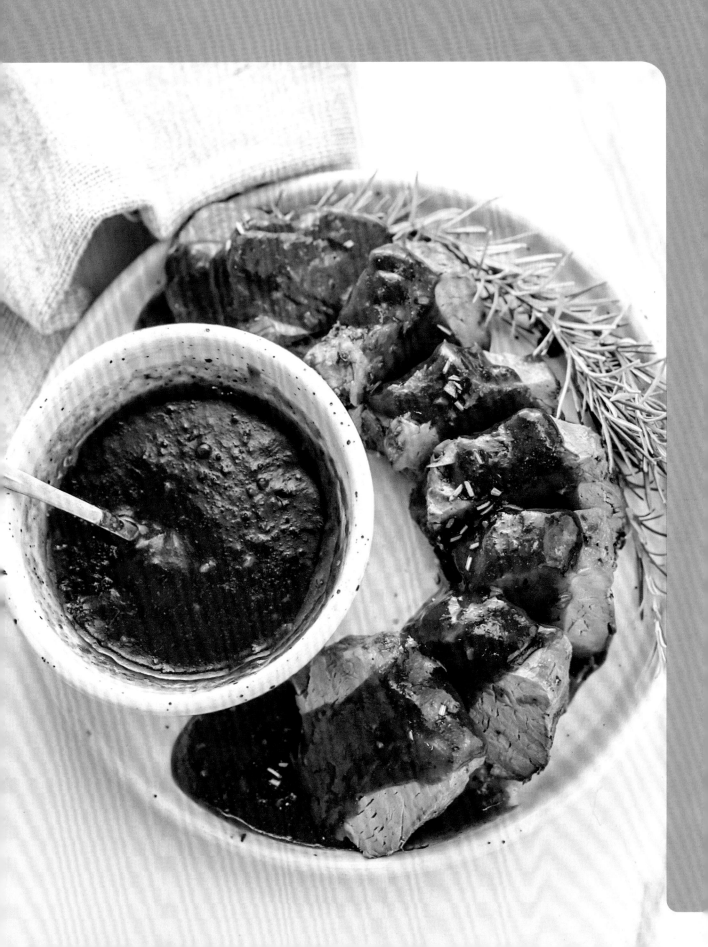

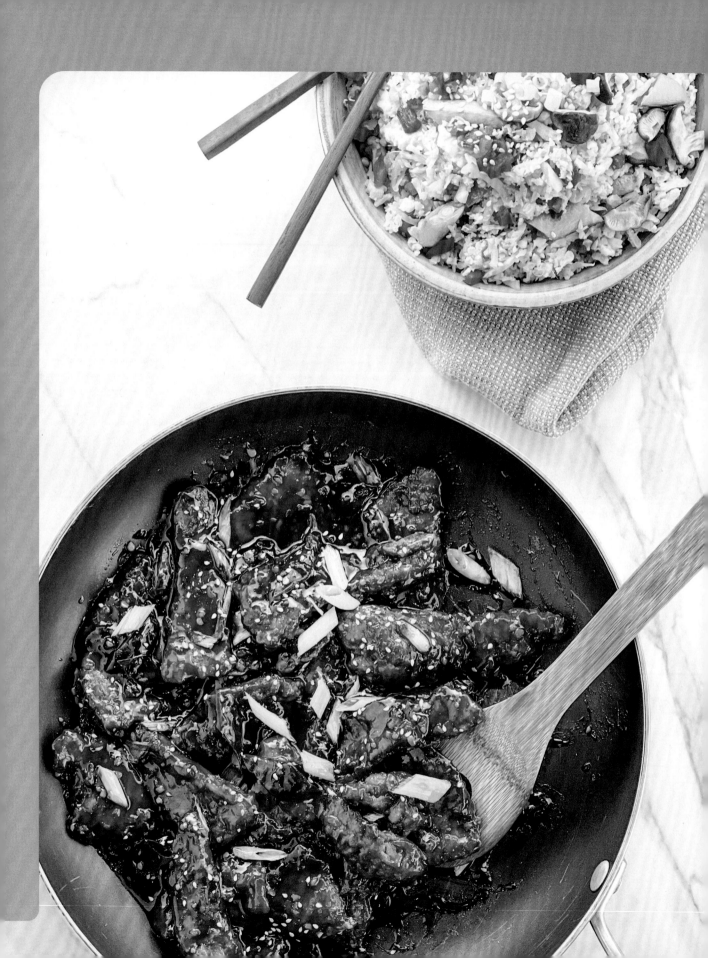

Crispy Sweet Mongolian Beef Ⓟ Ⓜ

Per serving: Calories: 496 Fat: 29g Net Carb: 19g (15%) Protein: 33g

Makes 4 servings | Prep time: 10 minutes | Cook time: 15 minutes

In a large bowl, whisk together 2 tablespoons of cornstarch, 1 tablespoon of oil, and the coconut aminos. Add the beef and toss well to coat. Cover and refrigerate for 1 hour.

Put the remaining ¼ cup of cornstarch in a shallow bowl. Dredge the beef in the cornstarch.

Heat the remaining ⅓ cup of oil in a large skillet or wok over high heat. Add the beef in a single layer and cook undisturbed for 1 minute, until seared. Flip the beef and sear the other side, about 1 more minute. Transfer the beef to a colander in the sink, allowing the excess oil to drain.

Return the skillet to medium heat. Add the garlic and ginger and cook until fragrant, about 2 minutes. Add the bone broth and bring to a simmer. Stir in the Swerve, coconut aminos, and red chiles. Simmer for 3 minutes. In a small bowl, whisk together the cornstarch and water, then whisk the mixture into the sauce in the skillet. Cook until the sauce has thickened, about 3 minutes. Add the beef and about three-quarters of the green onions. Mix and cook until all of the sauce is incorporated. Top with the remaining green onions and the sesame seeds.

Beef
¼ cup plus 2 tablespoons cornstarch or arrowroot powder, divided

⅓ cup plus 1 tablespoon avocado oil, divided

1 tablespoon coconut aminos or soy sauce

1 pound flank steak, sliced ¼ inch thick against the grain

½ cup chopped green onions, divided

½ teaspoon sesame seeds, for garnish

Sauce
1 tablespoon minced garlic

1 tablespoon minced fresh ginger

½ cup bone broth

2 tablespoons brown Swerve

½ cup coconut aminos or soy sauce

4 dried red chiles, sliced

2 tablespoons cornstarch or arrowroot powder

1 tablespoon water

Smoky Spiced Brisket ⓡ ⓟ ⓜ

Per serving: Calories: 425 Fat: 20g Net Carb: 8g (8%) Protein: 48g
Makes 8 servings | **Prep time: 10 minutes** | **Cook time: 8½ hours**

Sauce
1 cup no-sugar-added
   ketchup
½ cup brown Swerve
⅓ cup apple cider vinegar
1 tablespoon minced garlic
1 tablespoon Worcestershire
   sauce
2 teaspoons black pepper
2 teaspoons ground mustard
2 teaspoons onion powder
1 teaspoon cayenne pepper
1 teaspoon liquid smoke

Rub
1 tablespoon brown Swerve
1 tablespoon smoked paprika
1 teaspoon ground cumin
1 teaspoon onion powder
1 teaspoon garlic powder
1 teaspoon ground mustard
1 teaspoon dried oregano
½ teaspoon black pepper
½ teaspoon cayenne pepper
1½ teaspoons salt

Brisket
4 pounds beef brisket
2 tablespoons olive oil
1 tablespoon cornstarch or
   arrowroot powder
2 tablespoons water

Tip: Got leftover brisket?
Consider making Kimchi and
Brisket Stir-Fry. Simply mix
sliced brisket and chopped
kimchi into the Stir-Fried Rice
recipe on page 213.

Combine all of the sauce ingredients in a slow cooker and mix well.

In a small bowl, combine all of the rub ingredients. Rub the mixture all over the brisket. Place the brisket in the slow cooker and spoon the sauce over it. Cover and cook on low for 8–10 hours, until the meat is tender and the internal temperature is 195 degrees F.

When the brisket is almost done, preheat the oven to 400 degrees F.

Transfer the brisket to a rimmed baking sheet. Drizzle with the olive oil and bake for 15 minutes to brown the top.

Meanwhile, transfer the sauce to a skillet. In a small bowl, whisk together the cornstarch and water, then whisk the mixture into the sauce in the skillet. Cook over low heat until thickened, about 5 minutes. Spread the sauce over the brisket and bake for another 10 minutes.

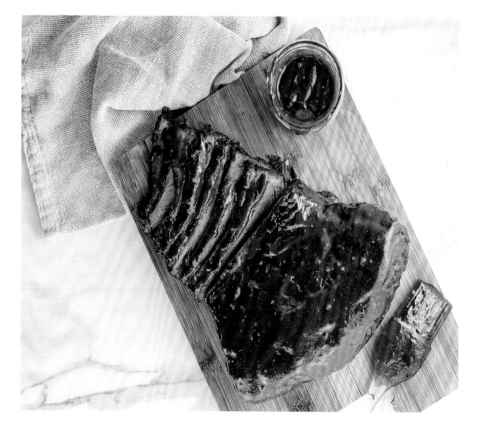

Grilled Sunday Steak 🅡 🅟 🅜

Per serving: Calories: 454 Fat: 29g Net Carb: 0g (0%) Protein: 45g
Makes 4 servings | **Prep time: 20 minutes, plus 3 hours to chill** | **Cook time: 10 minutes**

Pat the steaks dry with a paper towel, then sprinkle on both sides with the salt, pepper, paprika, and garlic powder. Cover with aluminum foil and refrigerate for 3 hours, then set aside at room temperature for 20 minutes before grilling.

Preheat a grill to high. For medium-rare steaks, sear for 1½ minutes per side, then reduce the heat to medium and grill for another 1½–2 minutes per side. If you prefer your steaks medium, add 1 more minute per side. Let the steaks sit for 5 minutes before serving.

4 (6-ounce) filets mignons
1 teaspoon kosher salt
½ teaspoon black pepper
½ teaspoon paprika
½ teaspoon garlic powder

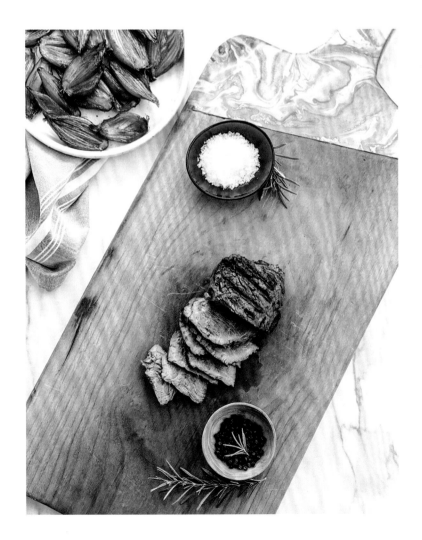

Fully Loaded Cheeseburger Skillet Ⓡ Ⓟ Ⓜ

Per serving: Calories: 459 Fat: 33g Net Carb: 3g (2%) Protein: 34g
Makes 6 servings | **Prep time: 20 minutes** | **Cook time: 15 minutes**

Thousand Island Dressing
¼ cup sour cream
3 tablespoons mayonnaise
2 tablespoons no-sugar-added ketchup
1 tablespoon minced pickles
1 teaspoon granular Swerve
½ teaspoon apple cider vinegar
¼ teaspoon onion powder
Pinch salt
Pinch black pepper

Beef
2 pounds ground beef
¼ cup finely chopped white onion
2 tablespoons no-sugar-added ketchup
1 tablespoon yellow mustard
1 teaspoon garlic powder
1 teaspoon onion powder
1 teaspoon salt
½ teaspoon black pepper
1½ cups shredded cheddar cheese, divided

Optional Toppings
Shredded iceberg lettuce
Pickle slices
Chopped red onion
Chopped tomatoes

In a small bowl, whisk together all of the dressing ingredients until smooth; set aside.

In a large bowl, combine the ground beef, onion, ketchup, mustard, garlic powder, onion powder, salt, and pepper and mix well. Heat a large skillet over medium-high heat and add the beef mixture. Cook, breaking it up, until no longer pink, about 12 minutes. Drain off any excess grease and liquid. Stir in ¾ cup of cheese. Remove from the heat and top with the remaining ¾ cup of cheese.

Drizzle with the dressing and serve with your favorite toppings.

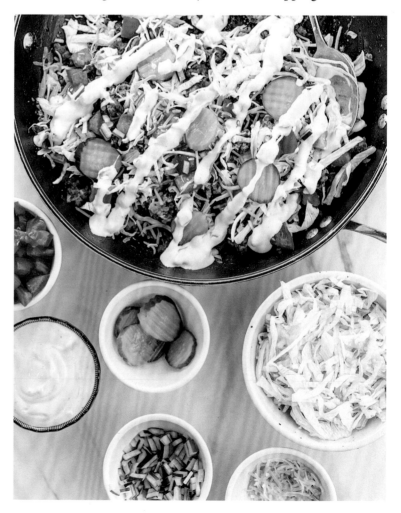

Creamy Swedish Meatballs ⓡ ⓟ ⓜ

Per serving: Calories: 571 Fat: 46g Net Carb: 6g (4%) Protein: 32g
Makes 6 servings | **Prep time: 20 minutes** | **Cook time: 25 minutes**

In a large bowl, combine all of the meatball ingredients (except the oil) and mix well. Shape into 1½-inch meatballs.

Heat the oil in a large skillet over medium-high heat. Add half of the meatballs and cook until browned on all sides and cooked through, about 15 minutes. Transfer the meatballs to a plate and repeat with the remaining meatballs.

Add the butter to any drippings remaining in the skillet and let it melt over medium-high heat. Meanwhile, in a small bowl, whisk together the cornstarch and water. Once the butter melts, add all of the sauce ingredients, including the cornstarch mixture, and whisk to combine. Simmer for 10 minutes. Return the meatballs to the skillet and toss to coat. Garnish with parsley.

Meatballs
1 pound ground beef
1 pound ground pork
¼ cup almond flour
¼ cup grated Parmesan cheese
2 large eggs, beaten
½ cup grated white onion
2 tablespoons minced fresh parsley, plus more for garnish
1 tablespoon minced garlic
2 teaspoons salt
½ teaspoon black pepper
½ teaspoon ground allspice
½ teaspoon ground nutmeg
1 tablespoon olive oil

Sauce
4 tablespoons (½ stick) unsalted butter
1 tablespoon cornstarch or arrowroot powder
2 tablespoons water
2 cups beef broth
½ cup heavy cream
¼ cup sour cream
1 tablespoon coconut flour
1 teaspoon stone-ground mustard
½ teaspoon salt
¼ teaspoon black pepper
¼ teaspoon ground allspice
¼ teaspoon ground nutmeg

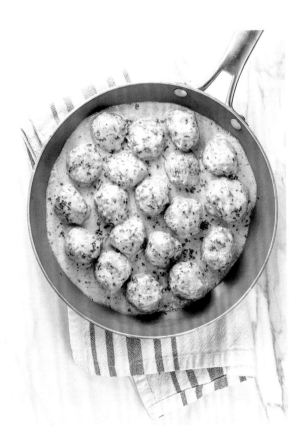

Hawaiian Meatballs and Spaghetti Squash Noodles P M

Per serving: Calories: 427 Fat: 27g Net Carb: 16g (14%) Protein: 21g
Makes 8 servings | **Prep time: 20 minutes** | **Cook time: 1 hour 15 minutes**

Meatballs

2 tablespoons olive oil, plus more for greasing
1 cup chopped yellow onion
1 teaspoon chopped garlic
1 tablespoon paprika
1 tablespoon five-spice powder
1 pound ground beef
1 pound ground pork
2 tablespoons almond flour
2 tablespoons grated Parmesan cheese, plus more for garnish
1 tablespoon minced fresh parsley, plus more for garnish
1 teaspoon salt

Pineapple Spaghetti Sauce and Squash

1 tablespoon olive oil
1 cup sliced red onion
1 cup sliced green bell pepper
¼ cup chopped fresh pineapple
1 (15-ounce) jar spaghetti sauce
2 spaghetti squash, cooked (see page 162)

Tip: If you serve the meatballs without the sauce and spaghetti squash, the dish drops down to 4% carbs.

Preheat the oven to 350 degrees F. Lightly grease a small baking pan with olive oil.

Heat the olive oil in a small skillet over medium heat. Add the onion, garlic, paprika, and five-spice and sauté until the onion is soft. Transfer the onion mixture to a large bowl and add the beef, pork, almond flour, Parmesan cheese, parsley, and salt. Mix until fully combined. Form about 28 meatballs the size of golf balls and place in the prepared baking pan. Bake for 25 minutes, or until cooked through.

To make the sauce, heat the olive oil in a large skillet over medium-high heat. Add the onion and bell pepper and sauté until soft, about 5 minutes. Add the pineapple and sauté for another 3 minutes. Add the spaghetti sauce and bring to a simmer.

Add the meatballs to the sauce and continue to simmer for another 10 minutes. Serve over the baked spaghetti squash, using the squash halves as bowls. Garnish with additional parsley and Parmesan cheese.

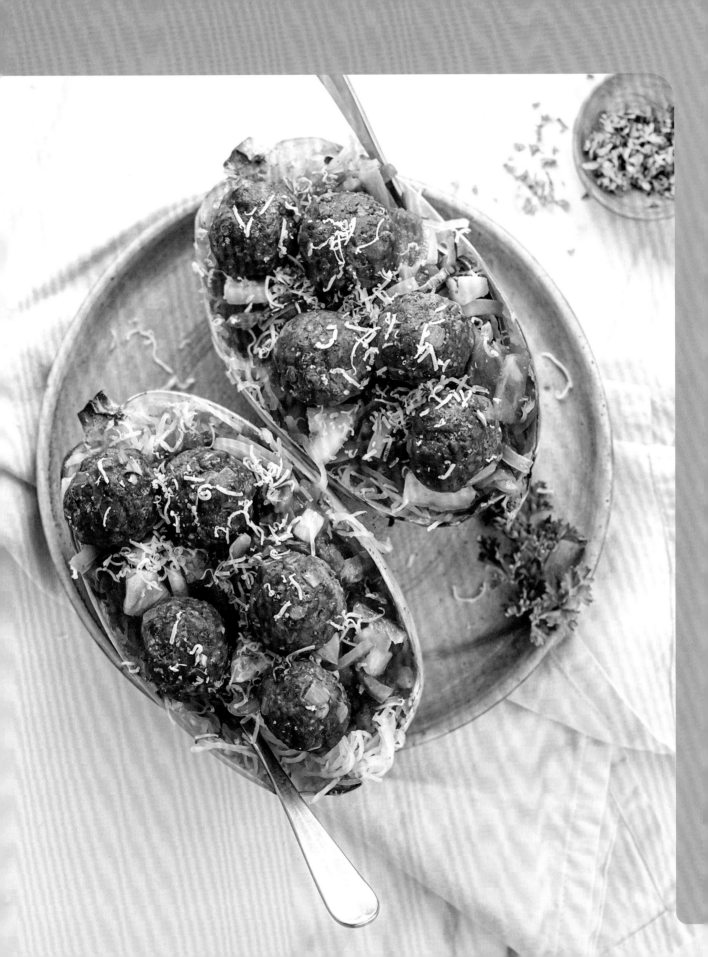

Glazed Sweet Onion Meatloaf ® ® ◉

Per serving: Calories: 400 Fat: 24g Net Carb: 9g (9%) Protein: 34g
Makes 6 servings | **Prep time: 15 minutes** | **Cook time: 1 hour**

Meatloaf
1 tablespoon olive oil
1 yellow onion
1 tablespoon minced garlic
2 pounds ground beef
2 large eggs
⅔ cup crushed pork rinds
⅓ cup whole milk
¼ cup no-added-sugar
    ketchup
2 tablespoons minced fresh
    parsley
2 teaspoons salt
1 teaspoon black pepper
1 teaspoon Italian seasoning
½ teaspoon paprika

Glaze
¾ cup no-sugar-added
    ketchup
2 tablespoons brown Swerve
2 teaspoons apple cider
    vinegar
1 teaspoon garlic powder
½ teaspoon onion powder
¼ teaspoon salt
¼ teaspoon black pepper

Preheat the oven to 375 degrees F. Line a 9 × 5-inch loaf pan with parchment paper.

In a small skillet, heat the olive oil over low heat. Add the onion and garlic and cook until translucent but not browned, about 3 minutes. Transfer to a large bowl and set aside to cool.

Add the remaining meatloaf ingredients to the bowl and mix well. Press the mixture into the prepared loaf pan. Bake for 40 minutes.

In a small bowl, combine all of the glaze ingredients and mix well. Spread the glaze over the meatloaf and bake for another 15 minutes, or until the internal temperature reaches 160 degrees F. Let rest for 10 minutes before slicing.

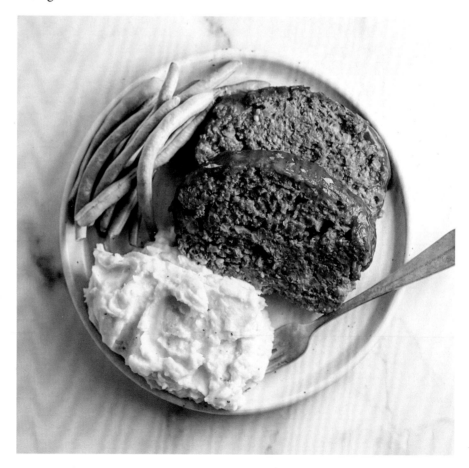

Spiced Beef Chili R P M

Per serving: Calories: 267 Fat: 15g Net Carb: 6g (9%) Protein: 22g
Makes 8 servings | **Prep time: 10 minutes** | **Cook time: 1 hour 45 minutes**

In a large pot, melt the butter over medium heat. Add the garlic, bell pepper, and onion and cook until tender, about 5 minutes. Add the beef and cook, breaking it up, until no longer pink, about 10 minutes. Add all of the remaining ingredients and stir well. Bring to a simmer, then turn the heat down to low and simmer for 1½ hours. Serve with your favorite toppings.

1 tablespoon unsalted butter
2 tablespoons minced garlic
1 cup minced red bell pepper
1 white onion, chopped
2 pounds ground beef
1 tablespoon chili powder
1 tablespoon smoked paprika
1 tablespoon unsweetened cocoa powder
½ teaspoon ground allspice
¼ teaspoon ground cloves
1 tablespoon ground cumin
1 tablespoon ground cinnamon
1 teaspoon salt
2 (14.5-ounce) cans diced tomatoes, undrained
1 tablespoon apple cider vinegar
½ cup beef broth
1 (4-ounce) can diced mild chiles, drained
Sour cream, for topping (optional)
Shredded cheddar cheese, for topping (optional)
Sliced green onions, for topping (optional)

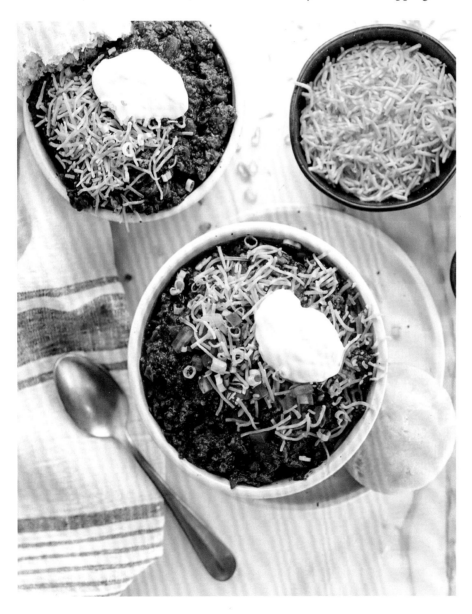

Tip: Another way to enjoy this chili is to make Chili-Stuffed Peppers! Preheat the oven to 400 degrees F. Cut the tops off 6 bell peppers and remove the seeds and ribs. Place the peppers cut side up in a baking pan and drizzle with avocado oil. Fill each pepper with chili and top with shredded cheddar cheese. Bake for about 30 minutes, until bubbly.

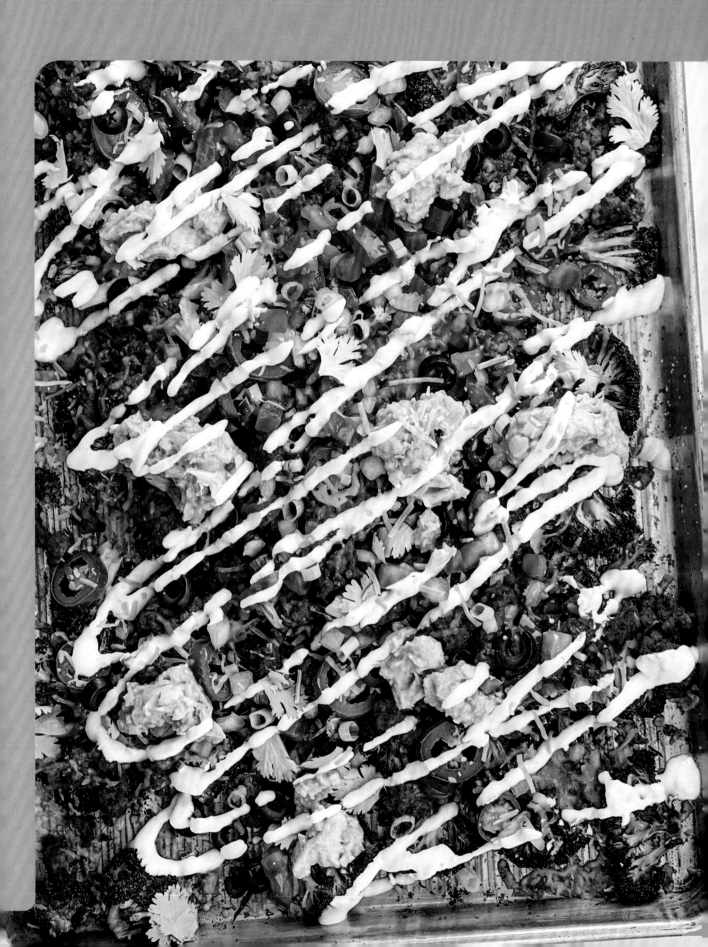

Crispy Loaded Brocco Nachos ⓟ ⓜ

Per serving: Calories: 334 Fat: 18g Net Carb: 8g (11%) Protein: 22g
Makes 6 servings | **Prep time: 15 minutes** | **Cook time: 25 minutes**

Preheat the oven to 450 degrees F. Lightly coat 2 rimmed baking sheets with avocado oil spray.

Cut the broccoli into florets, then slice each floret in half lengthwise. Put the florets in a large bowl and lightly spray with the avocado oil, then toss with garlic, salt, and pepper. Spread the florets evenly over the prepared baking sheets. Roast for 20 minutes, or until tender and charred.

Meanwhile, in a large skillet, cook the ground beef over medium heat, breaking it up, until no longer pink, about 10 minutes. Drain off any excess grease and liquid. Add the taco seasoning and water and simmer until the liquid has been absorbed, about 5 minutes.

Combine the broccoli florets on one baking sheet, spreading them out. Sprinkle the broccoli with the ground beef, cheese, jalapeños, olives, and onion. Return the sheet to the oven and bake for 5 minutes, or until the cheese has melted. Remove from the oven and top with the pico de gallo, guacamole, and cilantro.

In a small bowl, combine all of the ingredients for the sour cream sauce. Use a large spoon to drizzle the sauce over the nachos right before serving (or transfer to a piping bag).

Broccoli "Chips"
Avocado oil spray
2 heads broccoli
2 tablespoons minced garlic
Pinch salt
Pinch black pepper

Nachos
1 pound ground beef
2 tablespoons taco seasoning
¼ cup water
½ cup shredded cheddar cheese
¼ cup canned sliced jalapeños
¼ cup sliced black olives
2 tablespoons minced red onion
½ cup pico de gallo
½ cup guacamole
¼ cup chopped fresh cilantro

Sour Cream Sauce
¼ cup sour cream
1 tablespoon heavy cream
¼ teaspoon onion powder
¼ teaspoon garlic powder
⅛ teaspoon salt

Creamy Garlic Shrimp Ⓡ Ⓟ Ⓜ

Per serving: Calories: 402 Fat: 28g Net Carb: 5g (5%) Protein: 28g
Makes 6 servings | Prep time: 10 minutes | Cook time: 15 minutes

1 tablespoon olive oil
2 pounds large shrimp, peeled and deveined
½ teaspoon sea salt, plus more to taste
¼ teaspoon black pepper, plus more to taste
1 tablespoon unsalted butter
1 tablespoon minced garlic
½ cup dry white wine
1½ cups heavy cream
½ cup nutritional yeast or Parmesan cheese
2 tablespoons minced fresh parsley

Tip: Nutritional yeast imparts a cheesy flavor that works well in a creamy recipe like this, but if you aren't a fan or simply don't have any on hand, then swap it out for grated Parmesan cheese.

Heat the oil in a large skillet over medium-high heat. Add the shrimp, season with the salt and pepper, and cook, flipping once, until pink and cooked through, about 8 minutes. Transfer the shrimp to a plate.

Add the butter and garlic to the skillet and cook until fragrant, about 1 minute. Add the wine, scraping up any garlic that is stuck to the skillet. Bring the mixture to a simmer and cook until it is reduced by half, about 5 minutes.

Turn the heat down to low and stir in the cream. Bring the mixture to a simmer and stir in the nutritional yeast until creamy and smooth.

Return the shrimp to the pan and toss until covered with the sauce. Season with additional salt and pepper. Top with the minced parsley and serve immediately.

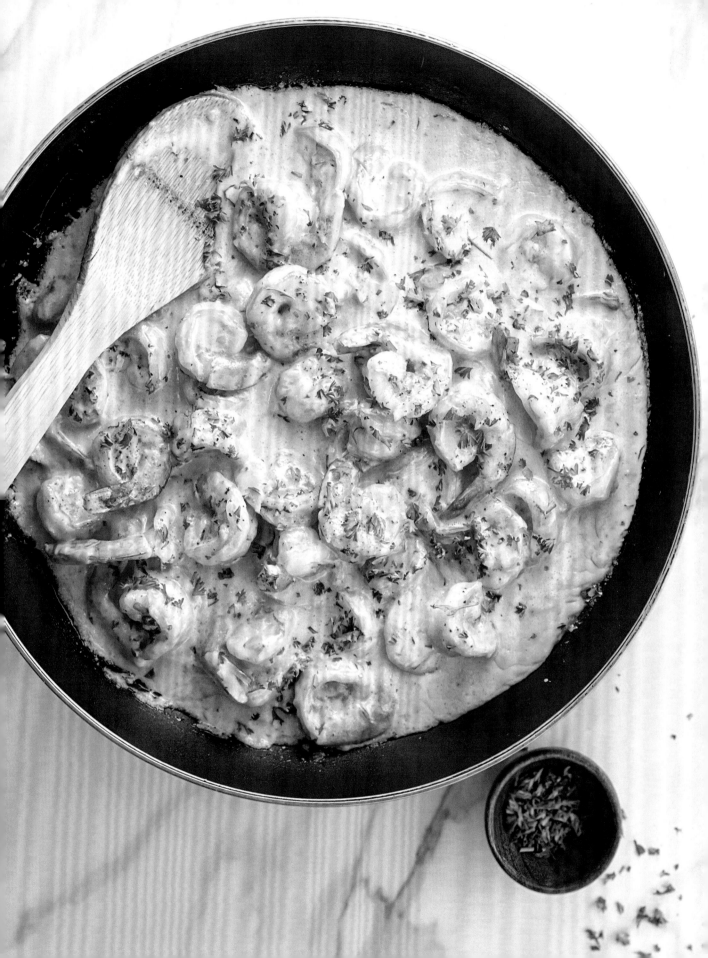

Seared Lemon Butter Scallops ⓡ ⓟ Ⓜ

Per serving: Calories: 256 Fat: 14g Net Carb: 7g (10%) Protein: 24g
Makes 4 servings | Prep time: 10 minutes | Cook time: 15 minutes

1 pound scallops
Salt and black pepper to taste
2 tablespoons avocado oil
2 tablespoons unsalted
  butter
1 tablespoon minced garlic
¼ cup dry white wine
1 teaspoon grated lemon zest
1 tablespoon lemon juice
2 tablespoons minced fresh
  parsley

Pat the scallops dry with paper towels, then season both sides with salt and pepper.

Heat the oil in a large skillet over medium-high heat. Add the scallops and cook, undisturbed, for 2–3 minutes per side, until seared and cooked through. Transfer the scallops to a plate.

Return the skillet to medium-high heat. Add the butter and garlic and cook until fragrant, about 1 minute. Add the wine, scraping up any garlic bits that are stuck to the skillet. Bring the mixture to a simmer and cook until it is reduced by half, about 5 minutes. Add the lemon zest and juice. Remove from the heat. Return the scallops to the pan and spoon the sauce over the scallops. Garnish with the parsley.

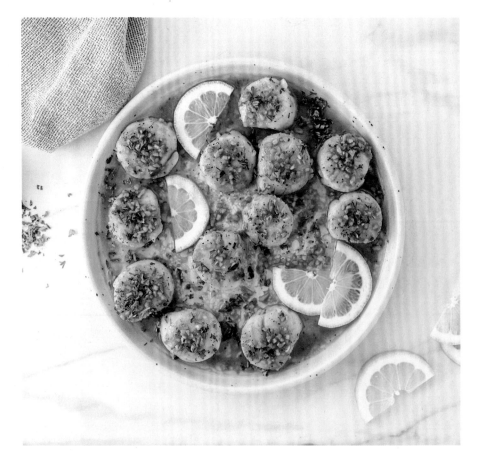

Sizzling Crab Cakes ⓡ ⓟ ⓜ

Per cake: Calories: 126 Fat: 9g Net Carb: 1g (3%) Protein: 9g
Makes 6 cakes | **Prep time: 10 minutes, plus 1 hour chilling time** | **Cook time: 10 minutes**

In a large bowl, combine the mayo, egg, mustard, Worcestershire sauce, Old Bay, lemon juice, celery, parsley, salt, and almond flour. Mix well. Stir in the crabmeat, being careful not to break it up. Form the crab mixture into 6 equal patties. Place on a parchment paper–lined plate, cover with plastic wrap, and refrigerate for 1 hour.

Heat the oil in a large skillet over medium-high heat. Add the crab cakes and cook for 4 minutes per side, until golden. Garnish with fresh parsley and serve with lemon wedges and your choice of sauce, if desired.

2 tablespoons mayonnaise
1 large egg
2 teaspoons Dijon mustard
2 teaspoons Worcestershire sauce
1 teaspoon Old Bay seasoning
1 teaspoon lemon juice
2 tablespoons finely diced celery
1 tablespoon minced fresh parsley, plus more for garnish
¼ teaspoon salt
¼ cup almond flour
8 ounces lump crabmeat, picked over
1 tablespoon avocado oil
Lemon wedges for serving
Creamy Adobo Sauce (page 199) or tartar sauce, for serving (optional)

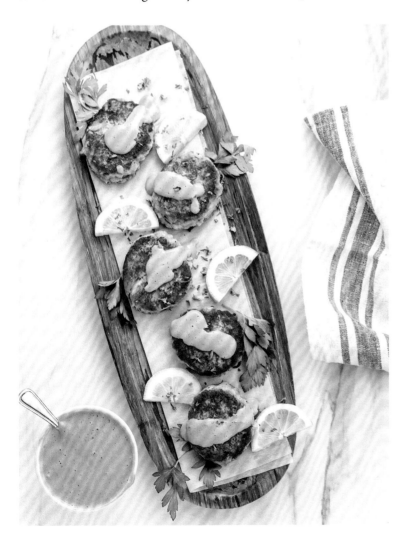

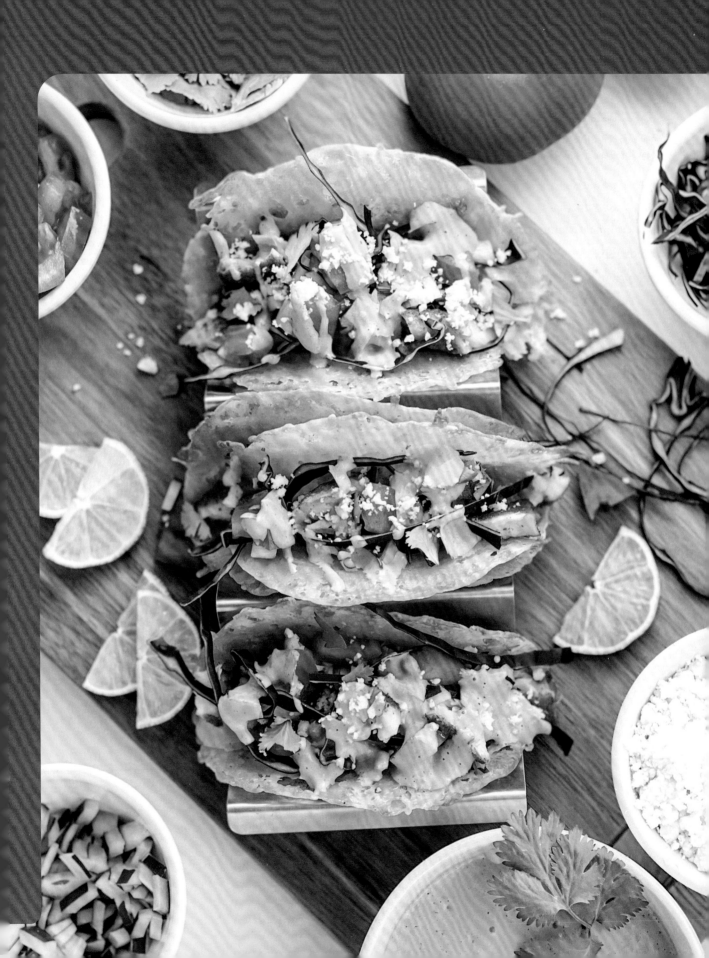

Baja Fish Tacos R P M

Per taco: Calories: 265 Fat: 20g Net Carb: 2g (3%) Protein: 18g
Makes 8 tacos | **Prep time: 15 minutes** | **Cook time: 35 minutes**

To make the taco shells, preheat the oven to 350 degrees F. Line a rimmed baking sheet with parchment paper.

Place the shredded cheese in eight ¼-cup mounds on the prepared baking sheet and flatten into circles. Bake for 5–7 minutes, until golden and browned on the edges. Increase the oven temperature to 375 degrees F.

Prop a wooden spoon with a rounded handle between 2 mugs, and lay a sheet of parchment paper over the spoon handle. Working 1 or 2 at a time, drape the cheese circles on the parchment so that they hang down and take on a crispy tortilla shell shape. Let cool for 5 minutes, until hardened, then transfer to a plate. Repeat with the remaining cheese circles.

To make the fish, replace the parchment paper on the baking sheet. Place the fillets on the parchment. In a small bowl, combine the cumin, cayenne, salt, and black pepper. Rub the spice mix into the fillets. Drizzle the fillets with the olive oil and top each with 1 teaspoon of butter. Bake for 20–25 minutes, until flaky.

Meanwhile, combine all of the sauce ingredients in a blender or food processor and blend until smooth.

Turn on the broiler and broil the fillets for 3 minutes, until golden. Divide the fillets between the taco shells and top with sauce and any of your favorite toppings.

Taco Shells and Fish
2 cups shredded cheddar cheese
2 (6-ounce) tilapia fillets
1 tablespoon ground cumin
½ teaspoon cayenne pepper
½ teaspoon salt
Pinch black pepper
2 (6-ounce) tilapia fillets
2 teaspoons olive oil
2 teaspoons unsalted butter, cut in half

Creamy Adobo Sauce
¼ cup mayonnaise
½ cup sour cream
¼ cup canned chipotles in adobo sauce
1 tablespoon lime juice
1 teaspoon garlic powder
1 teaspoon granular Swerve
¼ teaspoon sea salt

Optional Toppings
Lime slices
Chopped fresh cilantro
Shredded red cabbage
Minced red onion
Crumbled cotija cheese

Teriyaki Glazed Salmon 🅡 🅟 🅜

Per serving: Calories: 558 Fat: 36g Net Carb: 4g (3%) Protein: 50g
Makes 4 servings | **Prep time: 20 minutes** | **Cook time: 25 minutes**

Salmon
¼ cup salt
2 tablespoons granular Swerve
8 cups water
4 (8-ounce) skin-on salmon fillets
2 tablespoons avocado oil
Fresh thyme, for garnish (optional)

Teriyaki Glaze
1 teaspoon cornstarch or agar powder
1 tablespoon water
¼ cup soy sauce or coconut aminos
2 tablespoons lemon juice
2 tablespoons brown Swerve
1 tablespoon minced garlic
1 teaspoon salt

Preheat the oven to 300 degrees F.

In a large bowl, dissolve the salt and Swerve in the water. Add the fillets and set aside at room temperature for 15 minutes. Remove the fillets and pat dry with paper towels.

To make the glaze, in a medium bowl, whisk together the cornstarch and water. Add the soy sauce, lemon juice, Swerve, garlic, and salt and mix well.

Heat the oil in a large oven-safe skillet over medium-high heat. Add the fillets, skin side up, and cook until the flesh is browned, 2–3 minutes. Flip the fillets over and cover with the glaze. Transfer the skillet to the oven and bake for 15–20 minutes, until flaky and cooked through. Garnish with thyme, if desired.

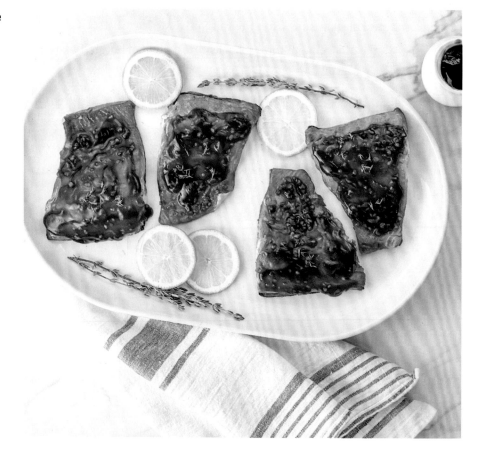

Herb-Roasted Halibut ⓇⓅⓂ

Per serving: Calories: 380 Fat: 8g Net Carb: 0g (0%) Protein: 72g
Makes 5 servings | **Prep time: 10 minutes** | **Cook time: 20 minutes**

Preheat the oven to 425 degrees F. Lightly grease a baking pan.

Place the fillets in the prepared pan and drizzle with the avocado oil. Sprinkle each fillet with the minced garlic, lemon zest, and marjoram and season with salt and pepper. Top each fillet with a slice of lemon. Roast for 15–20 minutes, until flaky and cooked through. Cover with aluminum foil if the tops are getting too dark before the fillets are cooked through.

5 (6-ounce) skin-on halibut
   fillets
1 tablespoon avocado oil
2 teaspoons minced garlic
1 teaspoon grated lemon zest
2 teaspoons dried marjoram
Salt and black pepper to taste
1 lemon, cut into 5 thin slices

Tip: This recipe is also great with skin-on salmon fillets!

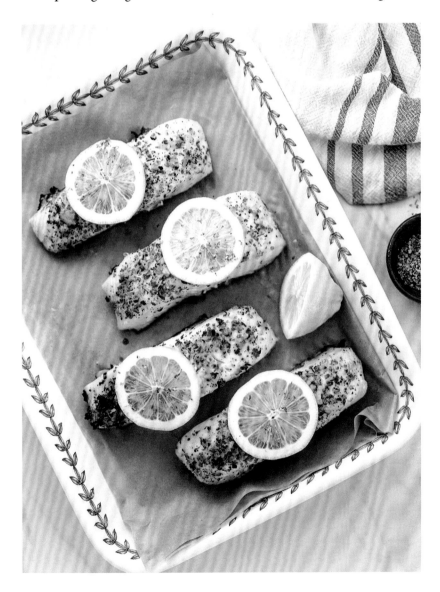

Baked Mac and Cheese Ⓡ Ⓟ Ⓜ

Per serving: Calories: 430 Fat: 36g Net Carb: 7g (6%) Protein: 19g
Makes 8 servings | **Prep time: 15 minutes** | **Cook time: 30 minutes**

8 ounces low-carb elbow pasta

1 teaspoon olive oil

4 tablespoons (½ stick) unsalted butter

2 tablespoons coconut flour

½ teaspoon salt

¼ teaspoon black pepper

½ teaspoon ground mustard

¼ teaspoon paprika

¾ cup whole milk

1¼ cups heavy cream

2 cups shredded cheddar cheese

1 cup shredded Gruyère cheese

Minced fresh chives, for garnish (optional)

Tip: If you want to increase the protein in this recipe, feel free to mix in crumbled cooked bacon, shredded cooked chicken, or pulled pork.

Preheat the oven to 350 degrees F. Grease a 9 × 13-inch baking pan.

Cook the pasta for 1 minute less than the package instructions for al dente. Drain and return the pasta to the pot. Toss with the olive oil.

Melt the butter in a large skillet over medium-high heat. Add the coconut flour, whisking to combine. Stir in the salt, pepper, mustard, and paprika. Add the milk and then the heavy cream slowly, whisking with each addition. Remove from the heat.

In a large bowl, combine the cheeses. Stir 1 cup of cheese into the sauce, whisking until melted. Add another 1 cup of cheese, whisking until melted. Add the sauce to the pasta and mix well. Transfer the mixture to the prepared baking pan. Top with the remaining 1 cup of cheese. Bake for 15–20 minutes, until the cheese is melted and bubbly. Garnish with minced chives if desired and serve hot.

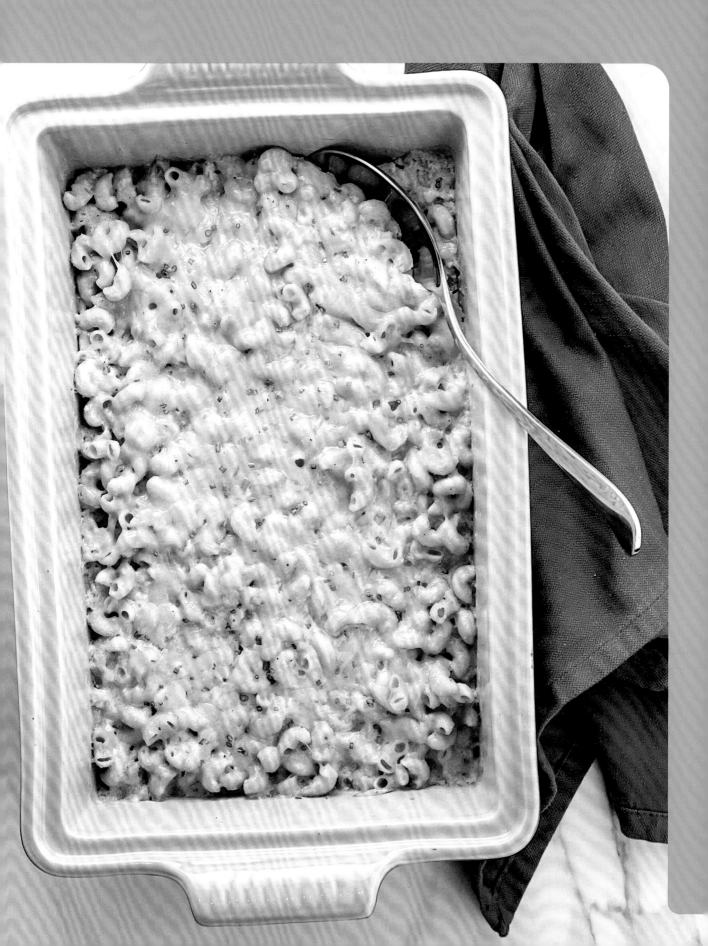

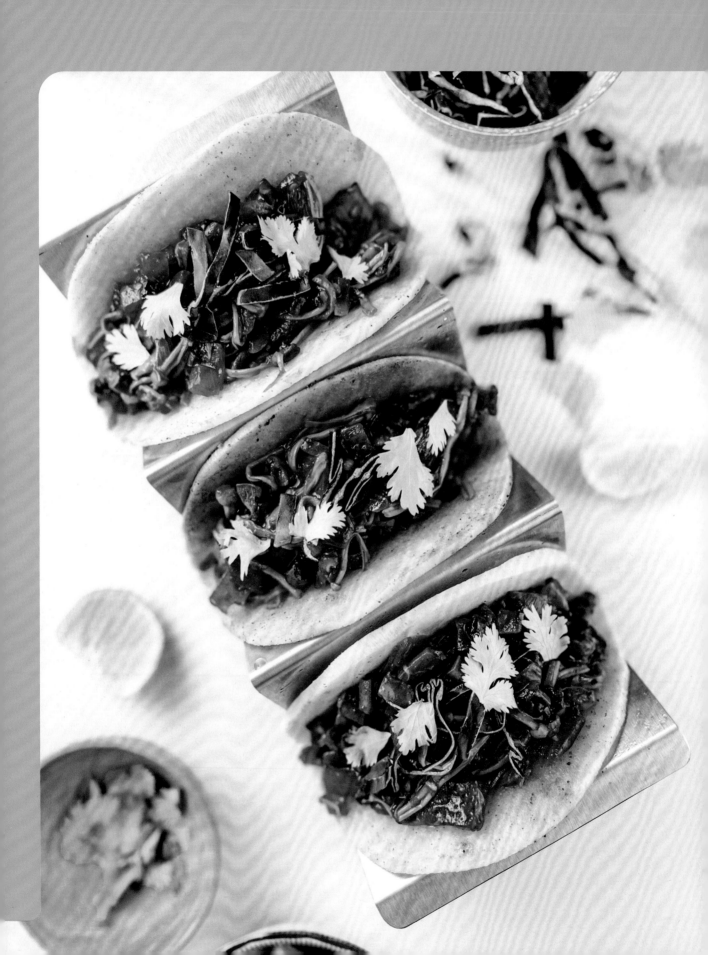

Adobo Braised Mushroom Tacos Ⓜ

Per serving: Calories: 524 Fat: 36g Net Carb: 25g (19%) Protein: 22g
Makes 2 servings | Prep time: 30 minutes | Cook time: 35 minutes

Heat 3 tablespoons of oil in a large skillet over medium-low heat. Add the onion and garlic and sauté for 4 minutes, until soft and fragrant. Add the cumin, paprika, coriander, tomato paste, and chipotle chiles in adobo. Mix well, turn the heat down to low, and cook for 5 minutes. Mix in the mushrooms, coconut aminos, broth, and Swerve, season with the salt and pepper, and cook, stirring occasionally, until the mushrooms are tender, about 20 minutes. If needed, splash the mushrooms with additional veggie broth to keep them moist and tender.

Heat the remaining 1 teaspoon of oil in a large skillet over medium-high heat. Add the jicama slices in a single layer and sprinkle with the smoked paprika. Cook for 1 minute, then flip and cook the other side for 1 minute. Transfer to a plate. Line the inside of each jicama "tortilla" with a slice of mozzarella cheese, fill each taco with the mushroom mixture, and top with cabbage and cilantro. Serve with lime slices for squeezing.

3 tablespoons plus 1 teaspoon olive oil, divided
1 white onion, diced
1 teaspoon minced garlic
1 teaspoon ground cumin
1 teaspoon smoked paprika
½ teaspoon ground coriander
1 teaspoon tomato paste
¼ cup canned chipotles in adobo, chopped
3 cups diced shiitake and/or button mushrooms
1 cup finely chopped enoki mushrooms
3 tablespoons coconut aminos or soy sauce
¼ cup vegetable broth, plus more as needed
1 teaspoon granular Swerve
¼ teaspoon sea salt
⅛ teaspoon black pepper
1 jicama, peeled and sliced into 6 thin rounds
¼ teaspoon smoked paprika
6 slices mozzarella cheese
¼ cup shredded red cabbage
¼ cup chopped fresh cilantro
Lime slices, for serving

Tip: Not feeling like tacos? These flavorful braised mushrooms are fantastic as a filling in your next omelet or tossed with low-carb pasta. Or make a savory version of the Fluffy Pancakes on page 128 by omitting the Swerve and vanilla, then serve each pancake topped with a spoonful of these incredible braised mushrooms and a fried egg!

White Garlic Lasagna with Tofu Ⓡ Ⓟ Ⓜ

Per serving: Calories: 482   Fat: 40g   Net Carb: 10g (8%)   Protein: 21g
Makes 8 servings | **Prep time: 30 minutes** | **Cook time: 45 minutes**

Lasagna Base

3 large zucchini, thinly sliced lengthwise

Salt to taste

12 ounces firm tofu, drained

2 cups shredded mozzarella cheese

Fresh basil leaves, for garnish

White Sauce

4 tablespoons (½ stick) unsalted butter

1 teaspoon minced garlic

2 tablespoons coconut flour

½ teaspoon salt

1½ cups heavy cream

4 ounces cream cheese

¼ cup grated Parmesan cheese

Ricotta Filling

1 (15-ounce) container whole-milk ricotta cheese

1 large egg

2 cups chopped fresh spinach

¼ cup chopped fresh basil

2 teaspoons garlic powder

1 tablespoon Italian seasoning

½ teaspoon salt

Preheat the oven to 400 degrees F. Line a rimmed baking sheet with parchment paper.

Sprinkle the zucchini slices with salt and let sit for 15 minutes. Blot the zucchini dry with paper towels. Spread out the zucchini on the prepared baking sheet and bake for 3 minutes, flip, and bake for another 3 minutes. Set aside; leave the oven on.

To make the white sauce, melt the butter in a large skillet over medium-low heat. Add the garlic and cook for 2 minutes, until fragrant. Mix in the coconut flour and salt and cook for 3 minutes. Whisk in the cream and bring to a simmer. Stir in the cream cheese and Parmesan cheese, whisking until melted. Remove the skillet from the heat.

To make the ricotta filling, in a medium bowl, combine all of the ricotta filling ingredients and mix until fully combined.

Coat an 8-inch baking pan with cooking spray. Spoon half of the sauce in the bottom of the pan. Place half of the zucchini over the sauce in a single layer. Spread half of the ricotta filling over the zucchini. Crumble half of the tofu over the filling. Top with half of the shredded mozzarella cheese. Repeat with the remaining sauce, zucchini, ricotta filling, tofu, and cheese. Bake for 30 minutes. Turn on the broiler and broil for 5 minutes, or until golden. Garnish with basil leaves.

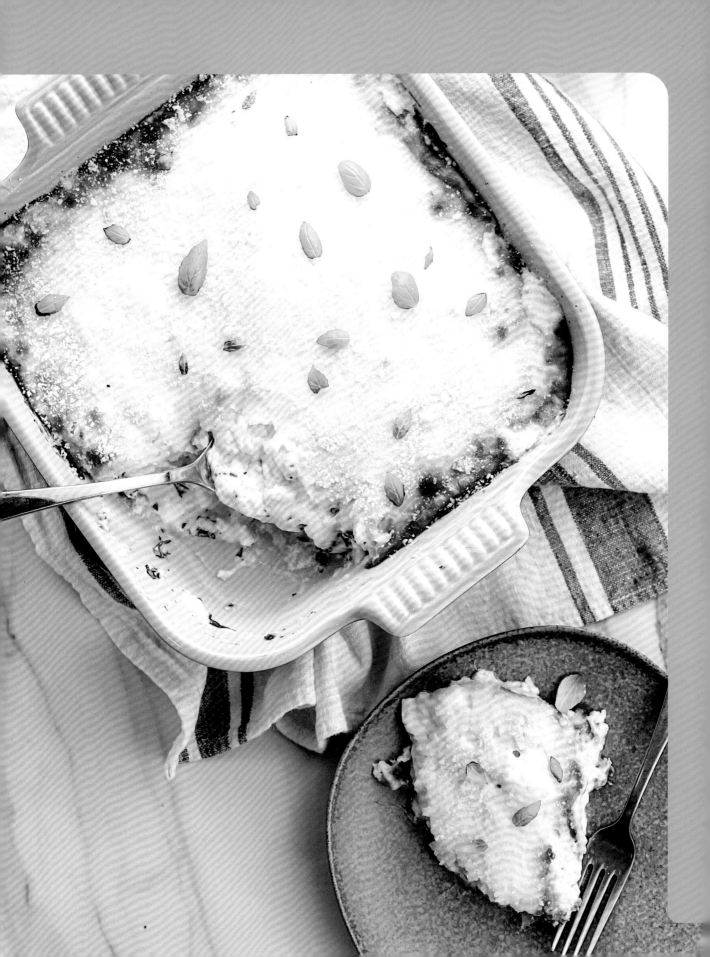

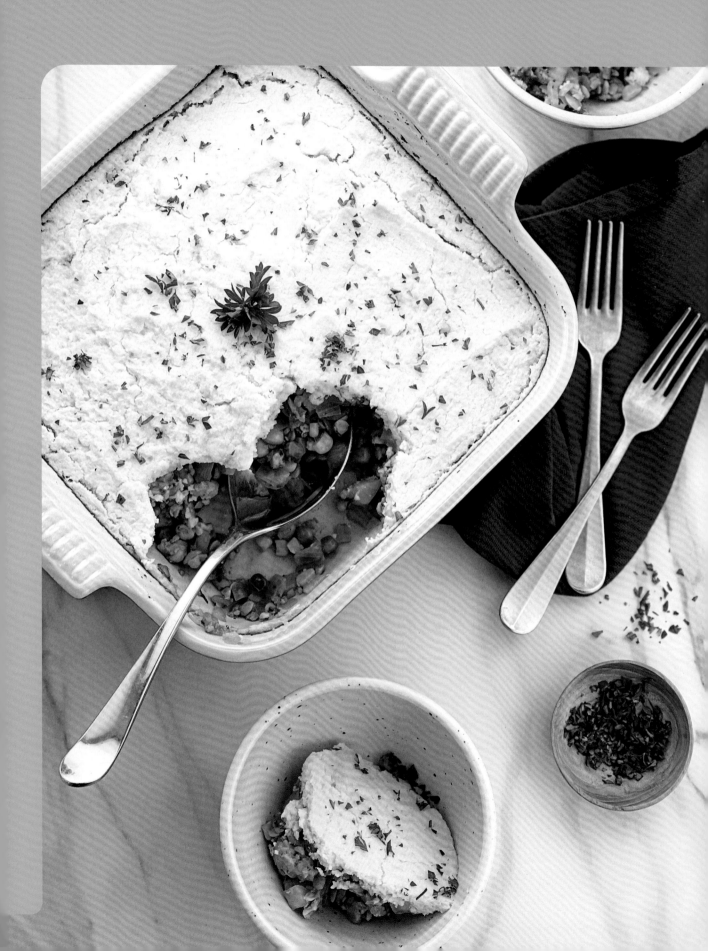

Tempeh Shepherd's Pie Ⓜ

Per serving: Calories: 322 Fat: 21g Net Carb: 15g (18%) Protein: 18g
Makes 4 servings | **Prep time: 20 minutes** | **Cook time: 45 minutes**

Preheat the oven to 400 degrees F. Lightly grease an 11 × 7-inch baking pan.

Pour an inch or so of water into a medium pot and add a steamer basket. Bring the water to a boil over medium-high heat and add the cauliflower and garlic cloves. Cover and steam until tender, about 10 minutes. Transfer the cauliflower and garlic cloves to a food processor, add the cream cheese, Parmesan, salt, and egg yolk, and blend until just smooth. Do not overblend.

Bring a shallow pot of water to a boil over medium-high heat. Add the tempeh and boil for 10 minutes. Drain and, when cool enough to handle, crumble the tempeh into small pieces.

Heat the oil in a large skillet over medium-high heat. Add the onion and garlic and cook until fragrant, about 3 minutes. Mix in the tempeh crumbles, tomato paste, broth, coconut aminos, rosemary, thyme, salt, and pepper. Simmer for 10–15 minutes, until thickened. Remove the skillet from the heat. Stir in the frozen peas and corn.

Spread the filling in the prepared baking pan. Spread the mashed cauliflower over the top, all the way to the edges. Bake for 20–25 minutes, until golden on top. Top with parsley.

Topping
1 head cauliflower, cut into florets
3 garlic cloves, peeled
¼ cup cream cheese
2 tablespoons shredded Parmesan cheese
¾ teaspoon salt
1 large egg yolk
1 tablespoon minced fresh parsley, for garnish

Tempeh Base
1 (8-ounce) package tempeh
2 tablespoons avocado oil
1 yellow onion, chopped
1 teaspoon minced garlic
2 tablespoons tomato paste
1 cup vegetable broth
1 teaspoon coconut aminos or soy sauce
1 teaspoon chopped fresh rosemary
1 teaspoon chopped fresh thyme
1 teaspoon salt
½ teaspoon black pepper
¼ cup frozen green peas
¼ cup frozen corn kernels

Soft Dinner Rolls Ⓡ Ⓟ Ⓜ

Per roll: Calories: 160 Fat: 12g Net Carb: 4g (10%) Protein: 15g
Makes 10 rolls | Prep time: 10 minutes | Bake time: 20 minutes

2 cups shredded mozzarella
    cheese
¼ cup sour cream
3 large eggs
1 cup almond flour
¼ cup coconut flour
1 teaspoon baking powder
¼ teaspoon baking soda
¼ teaspoon salt
1 tablespoon water
Flaky sea salt, for topping

Tip: These rolls are best served warm right out of the oven. Try to bake right before you plan to serve!

Preheat the oven to 400 degrees F. Line a rimmed baking sheet with parchment paper.

Pour about an inch of water into a small saucepan and bring to a simmer. Put the mozzarella cheese in a heatproof bowl and set it on top of the saucepan, making sure the bottom of the bowl does not touch the water below. Stir the mozzarella until fully melted, then transfer to a food processor. Add the sour cream, 2 eggs, almond flour, coconut flour, baking powder, baking soda, and salt. Pulse to combine.

Wet your hands and form ten 2-inch balls with the dough, then place on the prepared baking sheet. In a small bowl, whisk together the remaining egg and the water. Brush the egg wash over the rolls, then sprinkle with the flaky salt. Bake for 15 minutes. Turn on the broiler and broil for 3 minutes, or until golden.

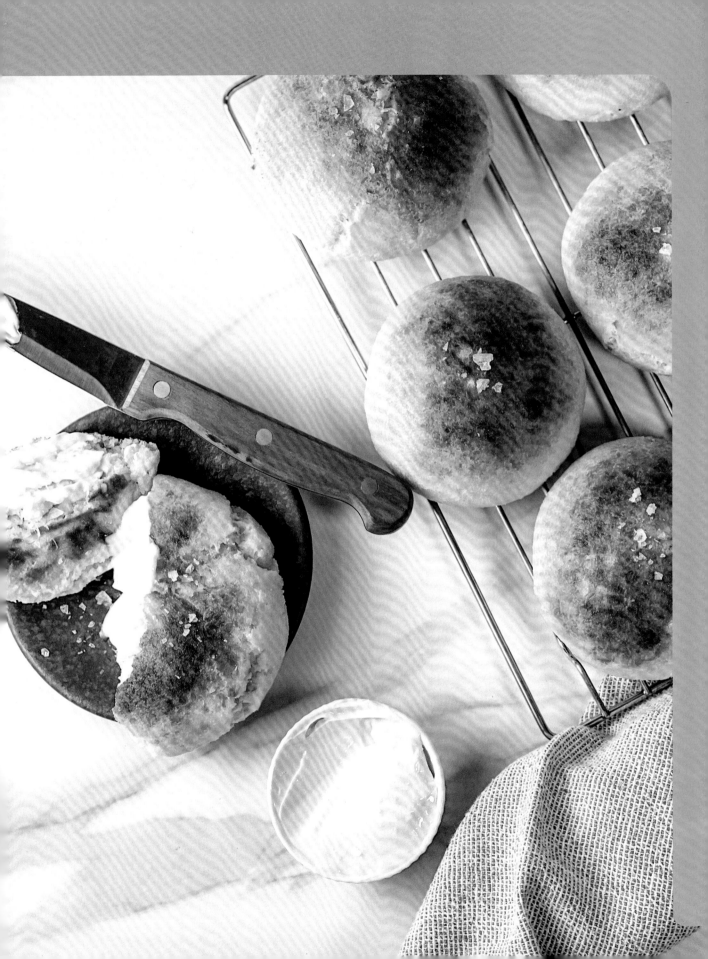

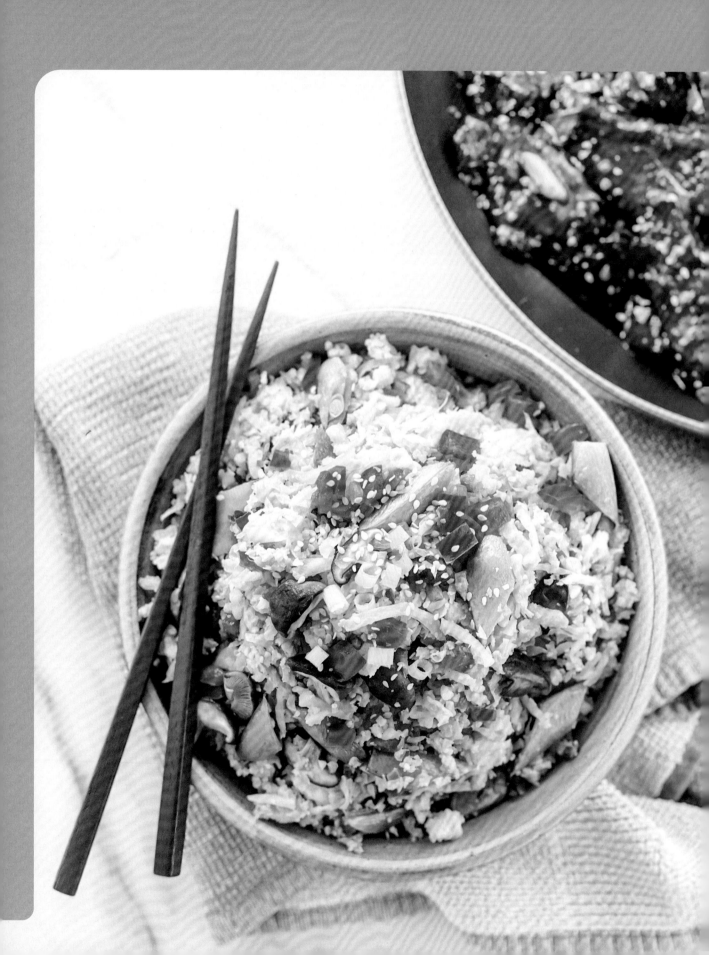

Stir-Fried Rice Ⓜ

Per serving: Calories: 235 Fat: 14g Net Carb: 11g (19%) Protein: 11g

Makes 4 servings | **Prep time: 20 minutes** | **Cook time: 30 minutes**

Bring a large pot of water to a boil. Add the cauliflower florets and cook for 5 minutes, then drain; wipe out the pot. Put the florets in a food processor fitted with the grating attachment and grate. Set aside.

Heat 1 tablespoon of avocado oil in the same pot over medium-high heat. Add the onion and bell pepper and sauté until tender, about 6 minutes. Add the snap peas and mushrooms and continue to cook for another 4 minutes. Transfer the veggies to a bowl and wipe out the pot.

Heat the remaining 1 tablespoon of avocado oil in the same pot over medium-high heat. Add the garlic and ginger and cook until fragrant, about 2 minutes. Add the grated cauliflower, stir, and cook for 4 minutes. Create a well in the center of the cauliflower rice and pour in the beaten eggs. Mix until fully incorporated with the cauliflower rice.

In a small bowl, whisk together the coconut aminos, sesame oil, and apple cider vinegar. Mix into the rice, then return the veggies to the pot. Season generously with salt and pepper and continue to cook for another 3 minutes. Top with green onions.

2 heads cauliflower, cut into florets

2 tablespoons avocado oil, divided

¼ cup diced red onion

1 red bell pepper, seeded and chopped

½ cup sliced snap peas (1-inch pieces)

1 cup sliced shiitake mushrooms

1 tablespoon minced garlic

1 tablespoon minced fresh ginger

2 large eggs, beaten

3 tablespoons coconut aminos or soy sauce

1 tablespoon toasted sesame oil

1 teaspoon apple cider vinegar

Salt and black pepper to taste

2 tablespoons sliced green onions

Tip: Want to save time? Feel free to use fresh or frozen cauliflower rice rather than steaming and grating your own.

Better-Than-Mashed-Potatoes 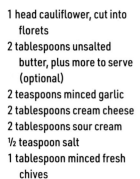 Ⓡ Ⓟ Ⓜ

Per serving: Calories: 117 Fat: 10g Net Carb: 3g (10%) Protein: 3g
Makes 4 servings | Prep time: 10 minutes | Cook time: 15 minutes

1 head cauliflower, cut into florets
2 tablespoons unsalted butter, plus more to serve (optional)
2 teaspoons minced garlic
2 tablespoons cream cheese
2 tablespoons sour cream
½ teaspoon salt
1 tablespoon minced fresh chives

Pour an inch or so of water into a medium pot and add a steamer basket. Bring the water to a boil over medium-high heat and add the cauliflower. Cover and steam until soft, about 10 minutes. Transfer the cauliflower to a food processor.

Melt the butter in a small skillet over medium heat. Add the garlic and cook until fragrant, about 2 minutes. Add the garlic and butter drippings to the food processor, along with the cream cheese, sour cream, and salt. Blend until smooth. Top with additional butter, if you like, and chives.

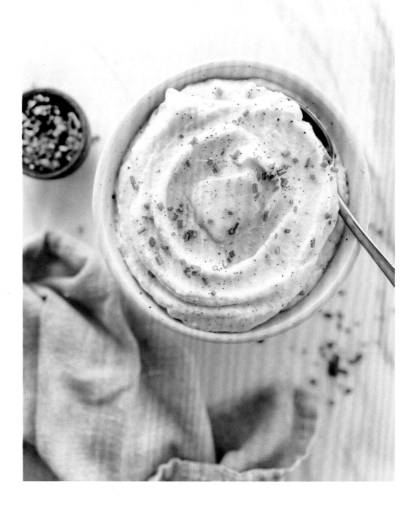

Caramelized Peppers and Onion Ⓜ

Per serving: Calories: 164 Fat: 14g Net Carb: 8g (19%) Protein: 1g
Makes 4 servings | **Prep time: 10 minutes** | **Cook time: 30 minutes**

Preheat the oven to 425 F. Lightly grease a rimmed baking sheet.

In a large bowl, toss the peppers and onion with the oil, salt, pepper, paprika, and thyme. Spread out on the prepared baking sheet and roast for 25–30 minutes, until tender and lightly charred. Toss with the lemon juice and parsley.

4 bell peppers (a mix of
   red, yellow, and orange),
   seeded and thinly sliced
1 red onion, thinly sliced
2 tablespoons avocado oil
½ teaspoon salt
¼ teaspoon black pepper
¼ teaspoon paprika
1 teaspoon chopped fresh
   thyme
1 tablespoon lemon juice
1 tablespoon minced fresh
   parsley

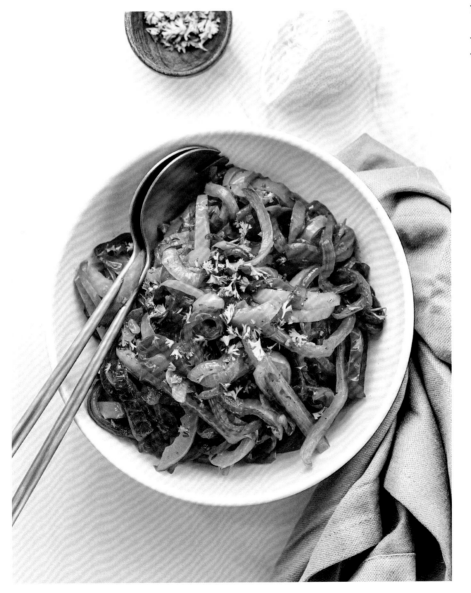

The Best Broccoli Ⓟ Ⓜ

Per serving: Calories: 251 Fat: 15g Net Carb: 9g (14%) Protein: 9g
Makes 4 servings | Prep time: 10 minutes | Cook time: 15 minutes

Olive oil spray
3 heads broccoli
¼ cup avocado oil
1 teaspoon minced garlic
Salt and black pepper to taste
½ teaspoon lemon juice
Grated Parmesan cheese, for
garnish (optional)

Preheat the oven to 450 degrees F. Lightly coat 2 rimmed baking sheets with olive oil spray.

Cut the broccoli into florets, then cut each floret in half lengthwise to create flat sides. Put the florets in a large bowl and toss with the avocado oil and garlic. Season with salt and pepper.

Spread the florets evenly over the prepared baking sheets. Roast for 10–15 minutes, until tender and charred. Sprinkle with the lemon juice and Parmesan, if desired, then toss and serve.

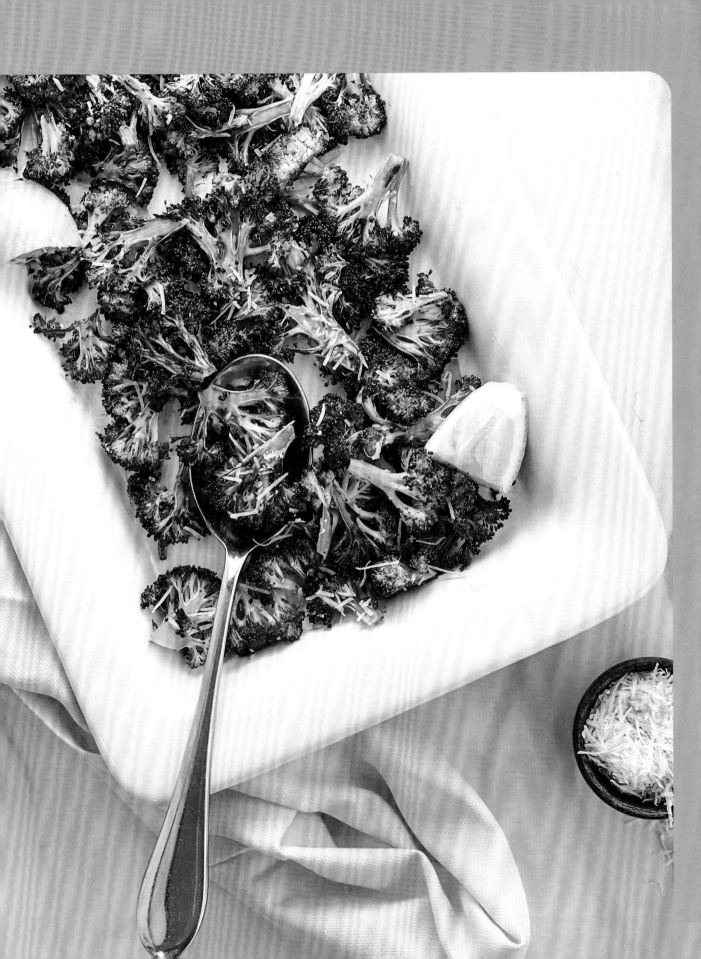

Favorite Noodles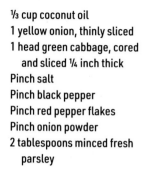

Per serving: Calories: 231 Fat: 17g Net Carb: 8g (20%) Protein: 4g
Makes 6 servings | **Prep time: 10 minutes** | **Cook time: 1 hour 15 minutes**

⅓ cup coconut oil
1 yellow onion, thinly sliced
1 head green cabbage, cored
   and sliced ¼ inch thick
Pinch salt
Pinch black pepper
Pinch red pepper flakes
Pinch onion powder
2 tablespoons minced fresh
   parsley

Preheat the oven to 250 degrees F.

Melt the coconut oil in a Dutch oven over medium heat. Add the onion and sauté until soft, about 4 minutes. Add the cabbage and mix to combine. Cook until the cabbage has wilted, about 5 minutes.

Cover the pot and transfer to the oven. Bake until the cabbage is very tender, about 1 hour, stirring once at the 30-minute mark.

Season the braised cabbage noodles with salt, black pepper, red pepper flakes, and onion powder and garnish with the parsley.

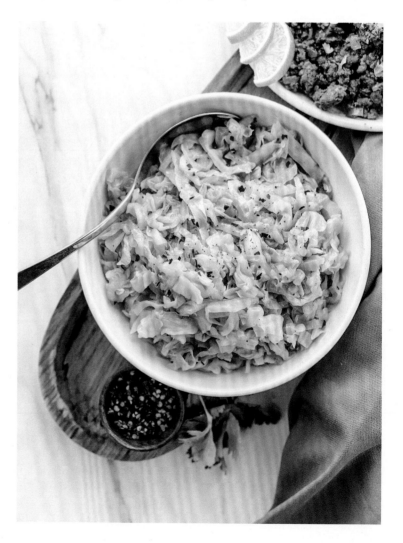

Herb-Sautéed Mushrooms ⓜ

Per serving: Calories: 169 Fat: 13g Net Carb: 7g (17%) Protein: 5g
Makes 4 servings | **Prep time: 10 minutes** | **Cook time: 15 minutes**

Heat a large skillet over medium-high heat. Add the mushrooms to the dry skillet, cut sides down. Cook for 4 minutes, until golden and seared. Flip the mushrooms and cook for another 2 minutes. Add the butter, garlic, salt, and pepper, stir, and cook until tender, about 5 minutes. Sprinkle with the parsley.

2 pounds mushrooms, cut in half
4 tablespoons (½ stick) unsalted butter
1 tablespoon minced garlic
½ teaspoon salt
¼ teaspoon black pepper
2 tablespoons minced fresh parsley

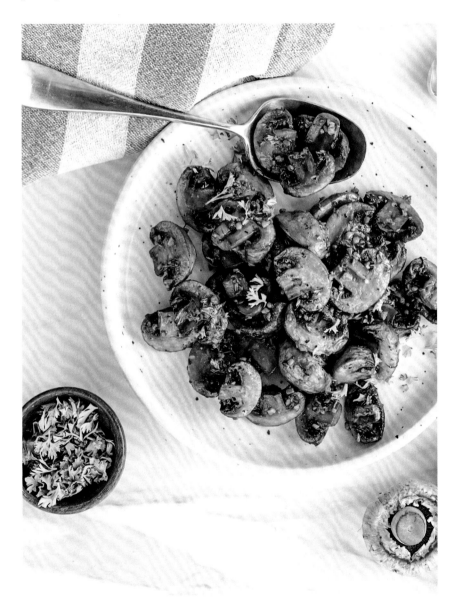

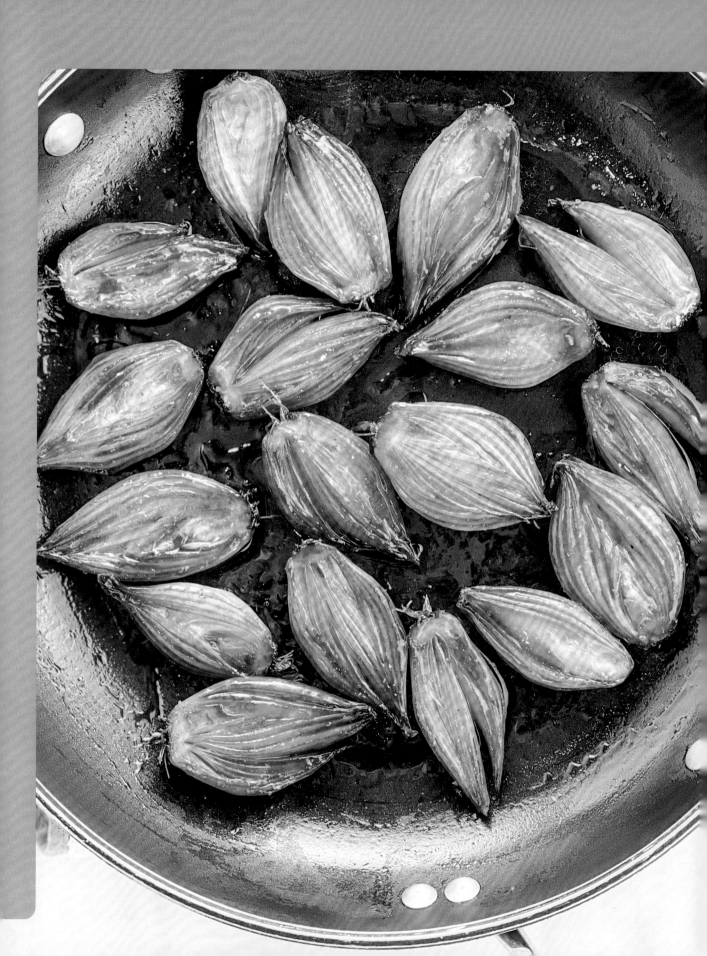

Melt-in-Your-Mouth Shallots ⓜ

Per serving: Calories: 185 Fat: 12g Net Carb: 10g (32%) Protein: 3g
Makes 6 servings | Prep time: 30 minutes | Cook time: 40 minutes

Put the shallots in a large bowl and cover with cold water. Soak for 20 minutes, then drain. Peel off the outer skins and cut the shallots in half, keeping the roots intact to keep the layers of each half together.

Preheat the oven to 250 degrees F.

Put the shallots in a large oven-safe skillet and just cover with water. Bring to a boil over medium heat. Reduce the heat and simmer for 5 minutes. Drain the shallots in a colander.

Wipe out the skillet. Melt the butter in the skillet over medium heat. Whisk in the Swerve, Worcestershire, and vinegar and bring to a low simmer. Add the shallots, cut sides down, turn the heat down to low, and cook for 20 minutes. Flip each shallot over, then transfer the skillet to the oven and roast for 10 minutes, until caramelized and tender. Season with salt and pepper to taste.

1 pound shallots (about 10)
4 tablespoons (½ stick) unsalted butter
1 tablespoon brown Swerve
1 tablespoon Worcestershire sauce
1 tablespoon balsamic vinegar
Salt and black pepper to taste

Cheesy Garlic Breadsticks Ⓡ Ⓟ Ⓜ

Per serving: Calories: 289 Fat: 25g Net Carb: 4g (5%) Protein: 9g
Makes 6 servings | **Prep time: 10 minutes** | **Bake time: 10 minutes**

Breadsticks
½ cup almond flour
3 tablespoons coconut flour
1 teaspoon garlic powder
1 teaspoon Italian seasoning
¼ teaspoon salt
½ cup sour cream
4 tablespoons (½ stick)
   unsalted butter
2 large eggs

Toppings
2 tablespoons unsalted
   butter, melted
½ teaspoon minced garlic
½ cup shredded mozzarella
   cheese, divided
⅓ cup grated Parmesan
   cheese
2 teaspoons minced fresh
   parsley
Flaky sea salt, for sprinkling
Tomato sauce, for serving
   (optional)

Preheat the oven to 425 degrees F. Line a rimmed baking sheet with parchment paper.

In a small bowl, sift together the almond flour, coconut flour, garlic powder, Italian seasoning, and salt.

In a medium bowl, beat the sour cream and butter together. Add the eggs one at a time, beating well to incorporate. Add the dry ingredients and mix well. Pour the batter onto the prepared baking sheet and use a spatula to spread the batter evenly into a large oval shape.

Mix the melted butter and garlic and drizzle over the batter. Sprinkle ¼ cup of mozzarella over the batter. Bake for 5 minutes. Sprinkle with the remaining ¼ cup of mozzarella and the Parmesan and bake for another 5 minutes. Sprinkle with the parsley and flaky sea salt and cut into 12 breadsticks. Enjoy warm, with tomato sauce for dipping, if you like.

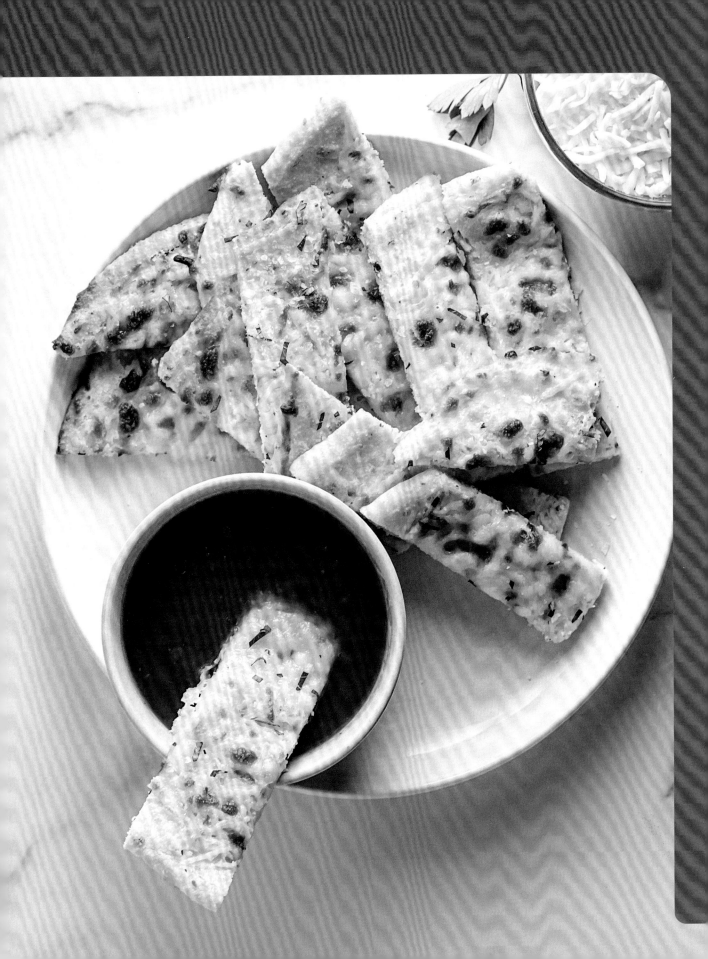

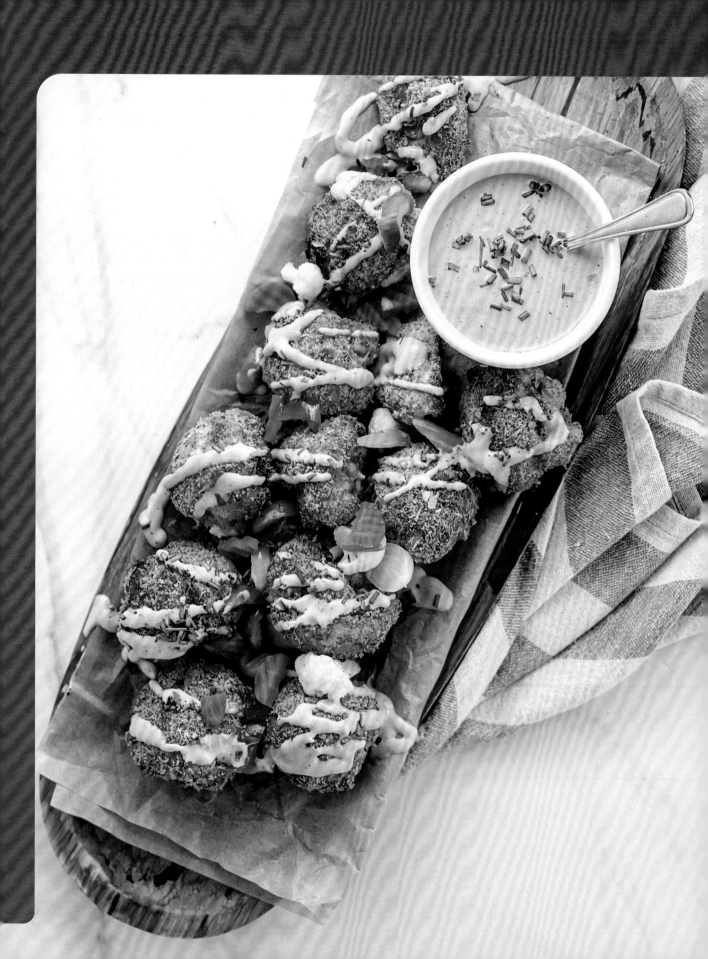

Crispy Breaded Cauliflower ⓡ ⓟ ⓜ

Per serving: Calories: 280 Fat: 20g Net Carb: 7g (10%) Protein: 15g
Makes 4 servings | **Prep time: 25 minutes** | **Cook time: 25 minutes**

Preheat the oven to 425 degrees F. Place a wire rack on a rimmed baking sheet. Coat the wire rack with cooking spray.

Bring a large pot of water to a boil over high heat. Add the whole head of cauliflower to the boiling water. Cover and cook for 5 minutes. Carefully remove the cauliflower and rinse with cold water. When it's cool enough to handle, quarter the cauliflower head, then separate each section into individual florets. Set aside.

In one shallow bowl, combine the coconut flour and garlic powder. In a second shallow bowl, whisk together the eggs, cream, and salt. In a third bowl, combine the almond flour, nutritional yeast, Parmesan, paprika, Italian seasoning, and cayenne.

Working in batches, coat the florets first in the coconut flour mixture, then in the egg mixture, and finally in the almond flour mixture. Arrange the florets, spaced ½ inch apart, on the prepared baking sheet. Roast for 15 minutes, or until crispy. Sprinkle with the pickled veggies and serve hot with Magic Sauce, if desired.

1 head cauliflower, trimmed
2 tablespoons coconut flour
¼ teaspoon garlic powder
2 large eggs
¼ cup heavy cream
½ teaspoon salt
½ cup blanched almond flour
2 tablespoons nutritional yeast
½ cup grated Parmesan cheese
1 teaspoon paprika
½ teaspoon Italian seasoning
Pinch cayenne pepper
1 (16-ounce) jar pickled carrots, cauliflower, celery, pearl onions, and red peppers, drained and chopped
Magic Sauce (page 135), for serving (optional)

Tip: This recipe works great in the air fryer. Preheat the air fryer to 370 degrees F and air-fry in batches for 9 to 12 minutes, until crispy.

Mini Pizzas Ⓡ Ⓟ Ⓜ

Per pizza: Calories: 73 Fat: 5g Net Carb: 2g (10%) Protein: 5g
Makes 12 pizzas | **Prep time: 10 minutes** | **Cook time: 20 minutes**

Crusts
1 cup cauliflower rice
1 teaspoon Italian seasoning
¼ teaspoon garlic powder
¼ teaspoon salt
1 cup shredded mozzarella
  cheese
2 large eggs
3 tablespoons almond flour
1 teaspoon coconut flour

Toppings
¼ cup marinara sauce
½ cup shredded mozzarella
  cheese
¼ cup mini pepperoni
Fresh basil leaves

Preheat the oven to 400 degrees F. Grease a 12-cup muffin tin.

In a medium bowl, combine the crust ingredients and mix well. Divide the mixture evenly among the 12 muffin cups, pressing it into the bottoms of the cups.

Bake for 12 minutes. Top each crust with 1 teaspoon of marinara sauce, a sprinkle of cheese, and a few mini pepperonis. Bake for another 8 minutes, until the cheese is melted. Top with basil and enjoy hot.

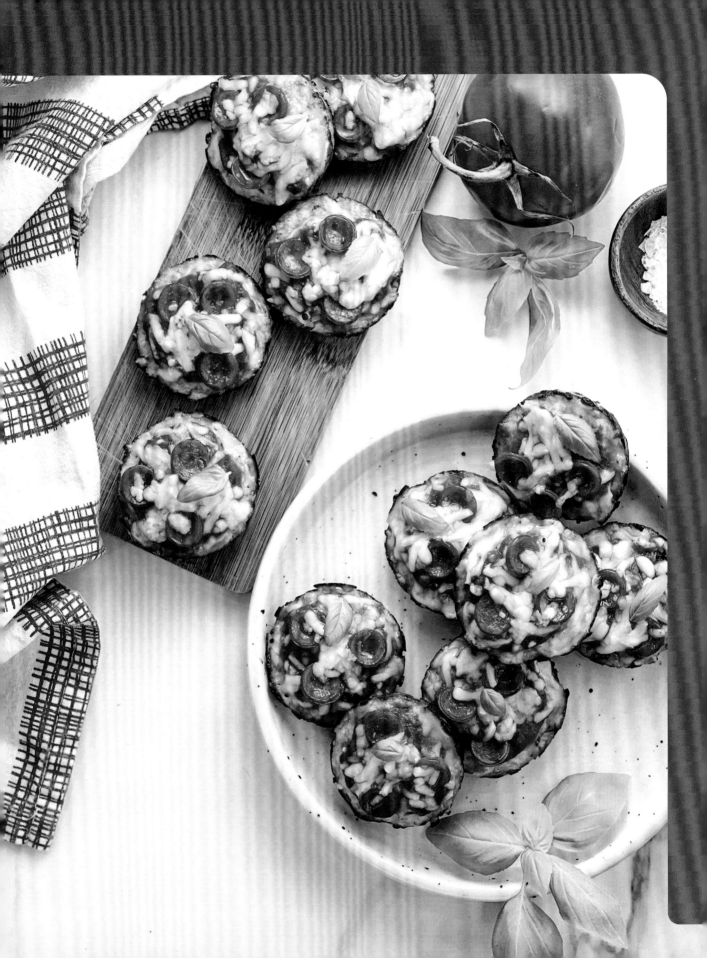

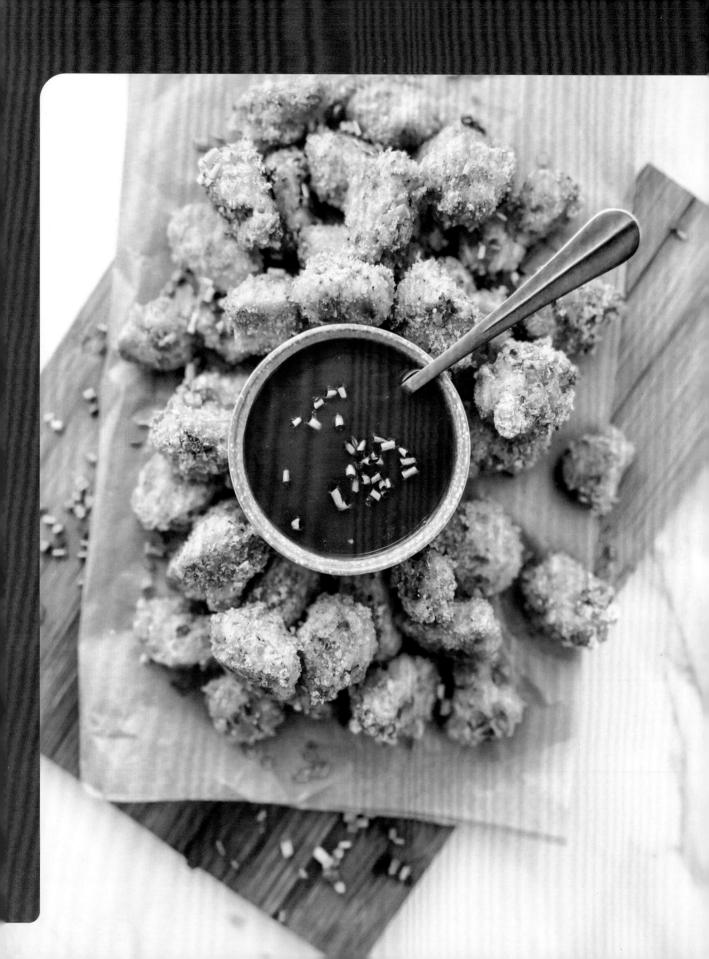

Baked Popcorn Chicken Ⓡ Ⓟ Ⓜ

Per serving: Calories: 340 Fat: 16g Net Carb: 3g (3%) Protein: 44g
Makes 4 servings | **Prep time: 10 minutes** | **Cook time: 20 minutes**

Preheat the oven to 425 degrees F. Line a rimmed baking sheet with parchment paper.

Combine the coconut flour, salt, pepper, garlic powder, and paprika in a large zip-top plastic bag. Add the chicken, seal the bag, and shake well to coat.

In one shallow bowl, whisk together the eggs and buttermilk. Put the crushed pork rinds in another shallow bowl.

Working in batches, coat the breaded chicken first in the egg mixture, then in the crushed pork rinds. Arrange the chicken, spaced ½ inch apart, on the prepared baking sheet. Bake for 10 minutes, flip the chicken, and bake for an additional 10 minutes. Serve with hot sauce for dipping, if desired.

⅓ cup coconut flour
½ teaspoon salt
½ teaspoon black pepper
½ teaspoon garlic powder
½ teaspoon paprika
3 large boneless, skinless chicken breasts, cut into bite-size pieces
2 large eggs
¼ cup buttermilk
1 (2.5-ounce) bag pork rinds, crushed into crumbs (about 1½ cups)
Hot sauce, for dipping (optional)

Tip: Pork rinds make a fantastic, low-carb replacement for panko bread crumbs. However, if you don't like pork rinds (or don't have any), feel free to replace them with the almond flour mixture ingredients used in Crispy Breaded Cauliflower (page 225).

Sweet Whipped Cream ⓡ ⓟ ⓜ

Per serving: Calories: 204 Fat: 22g Net Carb: 2g (4%) Protein: 2g
Makes 8 servings | Prep time: 20 minutes

1 pint cold heavy cream
6 tablespoons powdered
  Swerve, or more to taste
1 teaspoon vanilla extract
Pinch salt

Place the metal bowl and metal whisk attachment from an electric mixer in the freezer for 15 minutes. Combine all of the ingredients in the bowl and whisk on high until stiff peaks form, about 5 minutes. Serve and enjoy immediately!

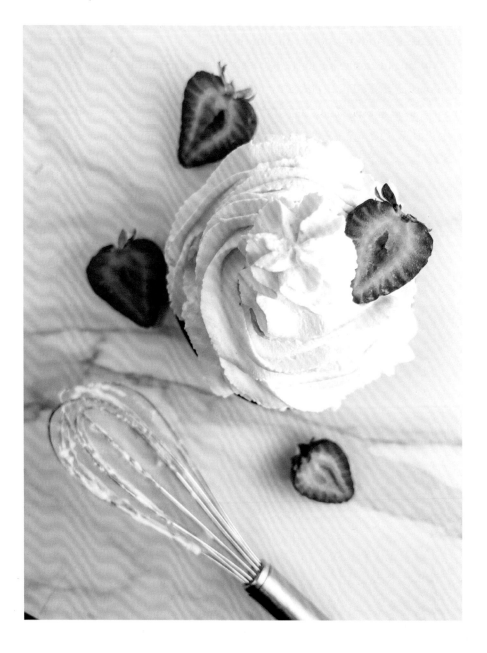

Cinnamon Roll Mug Cake 🅡 🅟 🅜

Per serving: Calories: 325 Fat: 26g Net Carb: 5g (6%) Protein: 21g
Makes 1 serving | **Prep time: 5 minutes** | **Cook time: 2 minutes**

Put the butter in a microwave-safe mug. Microwave for 20 seconds, until melted. Whisk the remaining mug cake ingredients into the butter and microwave for 1 minute.

In a small bowl, combine all of the frosting ingredients and mix well. Spread or pipe onto the hot mug cake. Enjoy immediately!

Mug Cake
1 tablespoon unsalted butter, melted
1 tablespoon coconut flour
1 tablespoon granular Swerve
½ teaspoon baking powder
Pinch salt
1 large egg, beaten
¼ teaspoon vanilla extract
½ teaspoon ground cinnamon

Cream Cheese Frosting
2 tablespoons vanilla protein powder
2 tablespoons confectioners Swerve
1 tablespoon cream cheese, room temperature
1 teaspoon whole milk, plus more as needed

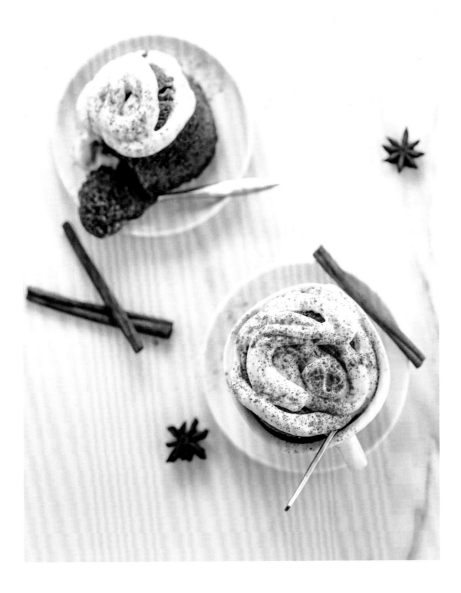

Tip: There are many ways to modify the flavors of your mug cake. Chocolate: Swap out the cinnamon for 1 tablespoon unsweetened cocoa powder. Funfetti: Omit the cinnamon, increase the vanilla to ½ teaspoon, and stir in a pinch of confetti sprinkles. Chocolate Chip: Omit the cinnamon, increase the vanilla to ½ teaspoon, and stir in 1 tablespoon stevia-sweetened chocolate chips.

Peanut Butter Chocolate Layered Mousse Ⓟ Ⓜ

Per serving: Calories: 540 Fat: 48g Net Carb: 20g (14%) Protein: 9g
Makes 6 servings | Prep time: 15 minutes, plus 30 minutes chilling time | Cook time: 5 minutes

Peanut Butter Mousse
½ cup peanut butter
4 ounces cream cheese, room temperature
⅓ cup confectioners Swerve
½ teaspoon vanilla extract
Pinch salt
½ cup heavy cream

Ganache
1 cup stevia-sweetened chocolate chips (such as Lily's)
1 cup heavy cream

Optional Toppings
Chopped peanuts
Flaky sea salt

With an electric mixer, beat together the peanut butter, cream cheese, Swerve, vanilla, and salt. In a separate bowl, beat the cream until stiff peaks form. Fold the whipped cream into the peanut butter mixture. Divide into 6 serving bowls. Chill in the refrigerator for 30 minutes.

To make the ganache, put the chocolate chips in a metal or heatproof glass bowl. Put the cream in a small saucepan and bring to a low simmer. Pour the cream over the chocolate and let it sit for 2 minutes. Stir until smooth. Pour the ganache over the peanut butter mousse. Serve immediately, topped with peanuts and flaky salt, or chill until serving.

Tip: If you love chocolate and peanut butter (and, ahem, who doesn't?), here's a recipe to try for Peanut Butter Mousse Brownie Pie. Bake the Frosted Fudge Brownies (page 236) in a pie pan at 350 degrees F for 20–25 minutes, until set. Cool completely. Spread the peanut butter mousse over the brownie pie and chill for 1 hour. Garnish with grated chocolate and chopped peanuts.

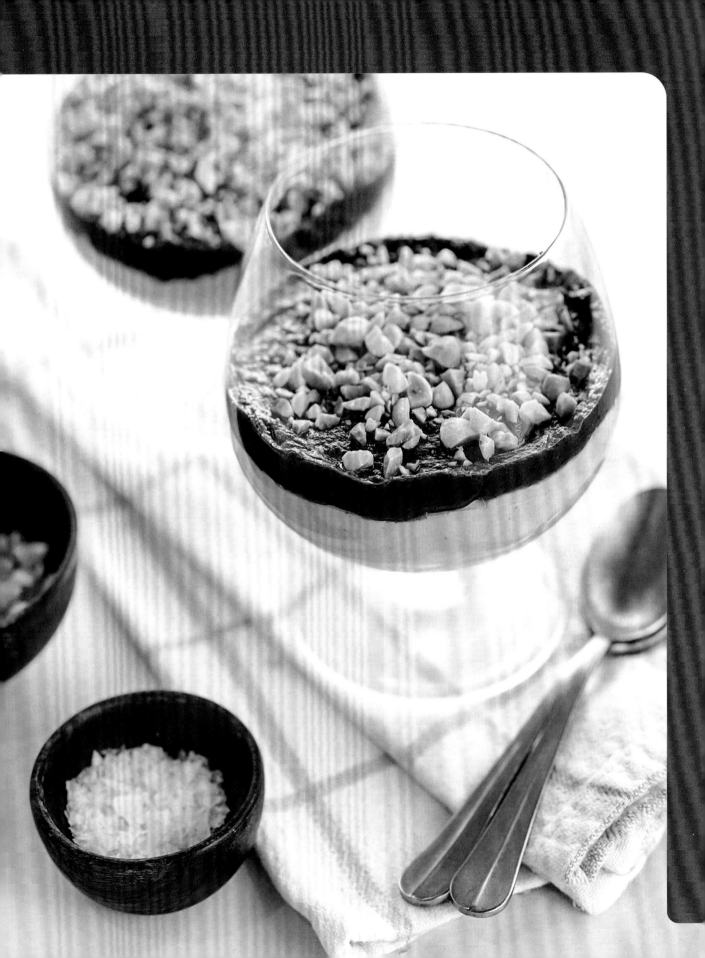

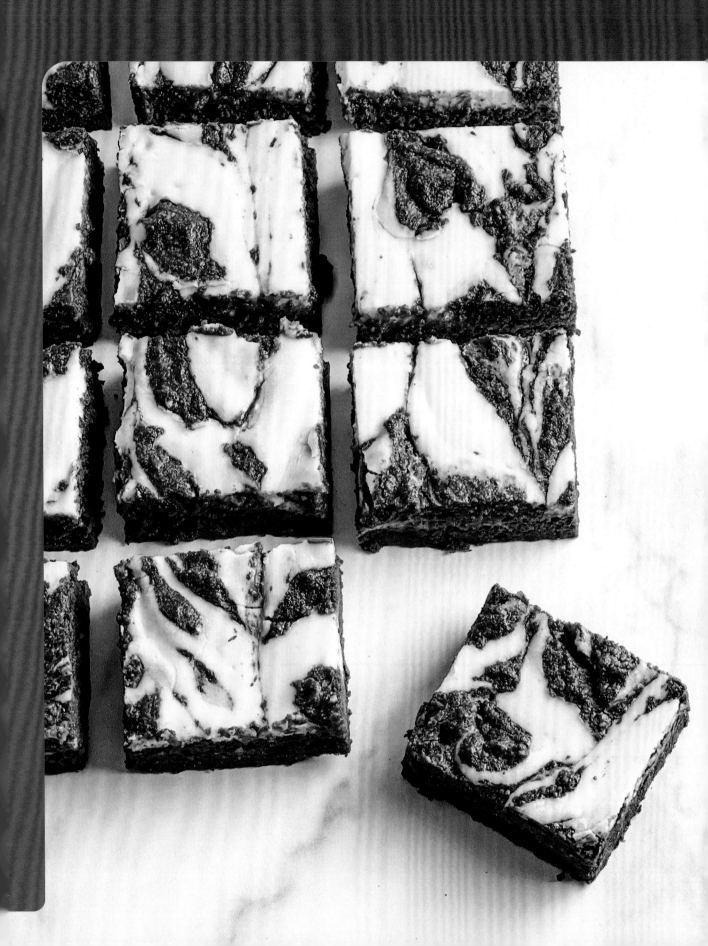

Swirled Cheesecake Brownies Ⓟ Ⓜ

Per serving: Calories: 175 Fat: 16g Net Carb: 5g (11%) Protein: 4g
Makes 20 servings | Prep time: 15 minutes | Bake time: 30 minutes

Preheat the oven to 350 degrees F. Line a 7 × 11-inch baking pan with parchment paper.

For the chocolate layer, pour about an inch of water into a small saucepan and bring to a simmer. Put the butter and chocolate chips in a heatproof bowl and set it on top of the saucepan, making sure the bottom of the bowl does not touch the water below. Stir the butter and chocolate together until melted and smooth. Remove the bowl from the heat. Mix in the cocoa powder, then the granular and brown Swerve, eggs and yolk (one at a time), vanilla, salt, and flour. Measure out ½ cup of the batter. Pour the rest into the prepared pan.

For the cheesecake layer: In the bowl of an electric mixer, beat the cream cheese and Swerve on medium speed until smooth. Add the egg and vanilla and beat until smooth. Pour the cream cheese mixture over the brownie mixture in the pan. Dot the top with the reserved batter. Use a butter knife to swirl the batter into the cream cheese layer to make a marbled effect. Bake for about 30 minutes, until the center has set. Cool completely before cutting and serving.

Chocolate Layer
12 tablespoons (1½ sticks) unsalted butter
½ cup sugar-free semisweet chocolate chips
½ cup unsweetened cocoa powder
1 cup granular Swerve
½ cup brown Swerve
2 large eggs plus 1 large egg yolk
1 teaspoon vanilla extract
½ teaspoon salt
1 cup almond flour

Cheesecake Layer
8 ounces cream cheese, room temperature
¼ cup granular Swerve
1 large egg
½ teaspoon vanilla extract

Frosted Fudge Brownies ⓡ ⓟ Ⓜ

Per serving: Calories: 180 Fat: 17g Net Carb: 2g (4%) Protein: 4g
Makes 16 servings | Prep time: 15 minutes | Bake time: 20 minutes

Brownies
1 cup almond flour
⅓ cup unsweetened cocoa
   powder
1 teaspoon baking powder
½ teaspoon salt
8 tablespoons (1 stick)
   unsalted butter, melted
2 large eggs
½ cup granular Swerve
1 teaspoon vanilla extract
½ cup plus 2 tablespoons
   chopped walnuts, divided

Frosting
8 ounces cream cheese, room
   temperature
½ cup unsweetened cocoa
   powder
4 tablespoons (½ stick)
   unsalted butter, room
   temperature
1 cup confectioners Swerve
1½ teaspoons vanilla extract
¼ cup heavy cream
Pinch salt
Flaky sea salt, for topping

Preheat the oven to 350 degrees F. Line a 7 × 11-inch baking pan with parchment paper.

In a medium bowl, whisk together the almond flour, cocoa powder, baking powder, and salt until smooth.

In a large bowl, combine the melted butter, eggs, granular Swerve, and vanilla and mix well. Add the dry ingredients and mix until just combined. Stir in ½ cup of chopped walnuts. Spread the brownie batter in the prepared pan. Bake for 20 minutes, until set. Let cool before frosting.

With an electric mixer, whip the cream cheese. Add the cocoa powder, butter, and confectioners Swerve. Scrape down the sides, add the vanilla, heavy cream, and salt, and whip until smooth. Spread the frosting over the cooled brownies. Sprinkle with flaky sea salt and the remaining 2 tablespoons of chopped walnuts.

Tip: I love the flavors of peppermint and chocolate around the holidays. To transform this recipe, swap out the chocolate frosting for a peppermint icing made by beating ½ cup room-temperature butter, 1 cup confectioners Swerve, 3 tablespoons heavy cream, ½ teaspoon vanilla extract, ½ teaspoon peppermint extract, and a pinch of salt. Cut the brownies and ice each one separately, allowing the white icing to drip down the sides. Top with crushed sugar-free candy canes or peppermint candies.

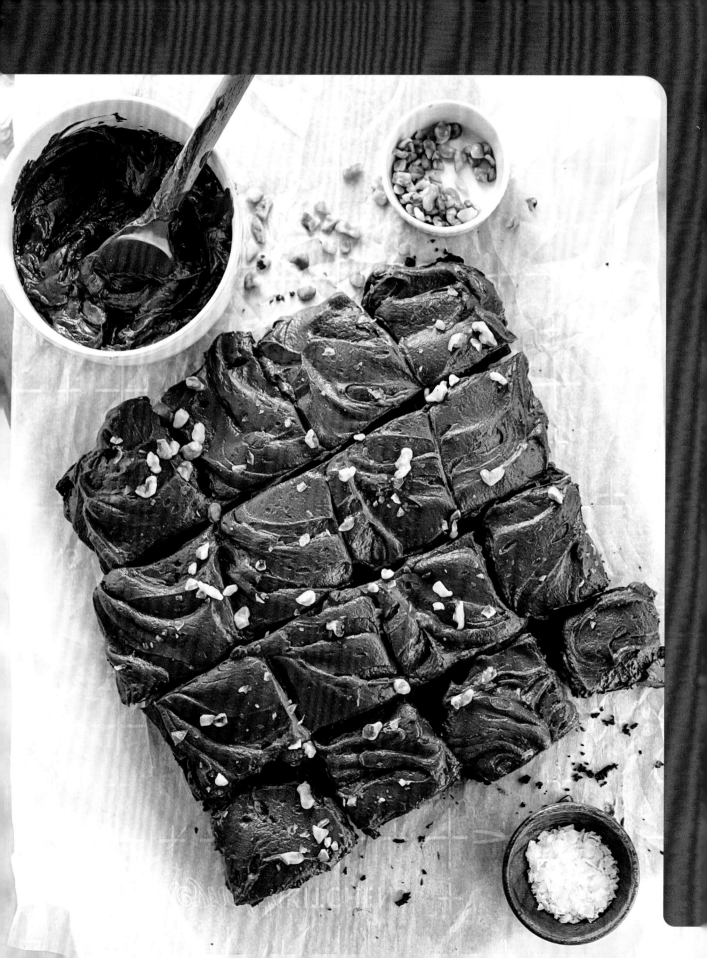

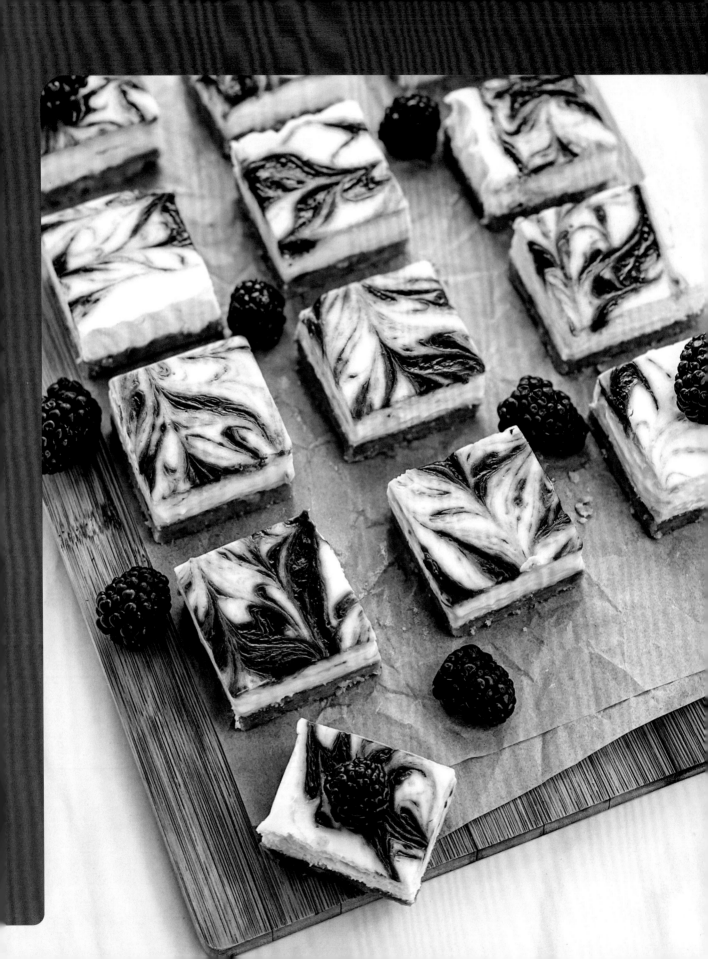

Blackberry Cheesecake Squares ® ℗ Ⓜ

Per serving: Calories: 255 Fat: 24g Net Carb: 4g (6%) Protein: 6g
Makes 16 servings | **Prep time: 20 minutes, plus 4 hours chilling time** | **Bake time: 35 minutes**

Preheat the oven to 300 degrees F. Line an 8-inch baking pan with parchment paper.

To make the crust, heat a large skillet over medium heat. Add the almond flour and toast until golden, stirring often, about 5 minutes. Transfer the almond flour to a large bowl, add the confectioners Swerve, cinnamon, salt, and melted butter, and mix well. Press the crust into the bottom of the prepared pan.

To make the blackberry sauce, in a small saucepan, combine 1½ cups of blackberries, 2 tablespoons of water, and the granular Swerve and cook over low heat until soft, about 10 minutes. Strain the sauce through a fine-mesh strainer to remove the seeds, then return the juice to the pan. In a small bowl, whisk together the cornstarch and remaining 1 tablespoon of water. Add the mixture to the juice and simmer over low heat until slightly thickened, about 3 minutes. Set aside to cool.

To make the cheesecake, using the paddle attachment of an electric mixer, beat the cream cheese and granular Swerve until smooth. Add the sour cream and vanilla and beat until smooth. Add the beaten eggs one at a time, beating until smooth. Add the lemon zest. Pour the batter over the crust and spread evenly. Spoon the blackberry sauce in dollops over the top of the cheesecake. Use a toothpick to swirl in and out of each dollop to create a design. Arrange the remaining ½ cup of blackberries over the top.

Bake for 30–35 min, until the middle is mostly set but still slightly wiggly. Turn off the oven, open the oven door, and let it sit for 25 minutes. Remove and cool to room temperature, then refrigerate for at least 4 hours before slicing and serving.

Crust
2 cups almond flour
¼ cup confectioners Swerve
1 teaspoon ground cinnamon
¼ teaspoon salt
8 tablespoons (1 stick) unsalted butter, melted

Blackberry Sauce
2 cups fresh or frozen blackberries, divided
3 tablespoons water, divided
1 teaspoon granular Swerve
1 teaspoon cornstarch

Cheesecake
16 ounces cream cheese, room temperature
½ cup granular Swerve
⅓ cup sour cream, room temperature
1 teaspoon vanilla extract
2 large eggs, room temperature, beaten
¼ teaspoon grated lemon zest

Tip: If blackberries aren't your favorite, feel free to omit the blackberry sauce and make New York-style cheesecake squares instead. Top with sliced fresh strawberries or a drizzle of the chocolate ganache on page 232.

Layered Caramel Cookie Bars Ⓡ Ⓟ Ⓜ

Per serving: Calories: 276 Fat: 27g Net Carb: 5g (7%) Protein: 4g
Makes 24 servings | **Prep time: 20 minutes** | **Bake time: 1 hour 15 minutes**

Caramel Cream
2½ cups heavy cream
4 tablespoons (½ stick)
  unsalted butter
1 cup brown Swerve
½ teaspoon vanilla extract

Sugar Cookie Crust
2 cups almond flour
¼ cup confectioners Swerve
1 teaspoon ground cinnamon
¼ teaspoon salt
8 tablespoons (1 stick)
  unsalted butter, melted

Toppings
1 cup stevia-sweetened milk
  chocolate chips (such as
  Lily's)
1 cup pecans, chopped
1 cup unsweetened shredded
  coconut

Tip: For more flavor, toast the pecans before using in this recipe!

Preheat the oven to 325 degrees F. Line a 7 × 11-inch baking pan with parchment paper.

To make the caramel cream, combine the cream, butter, brown Swerve, and vanilla in a medium skillet and bring to a boil over medium heat, stirring often. Turn the heat down to low and simmer, stirring occasionally, until thick and creamy but still liquid enough to pour, about 40 minutes.

To make the crust, heat a large skillet over medium heat. Add the almond flour and toast until golden, stirring often, about 5 minutes. Transfer the almond flour to a large bowl, add the confectioners Swerve, cinnamon, salt, and melted butter, and mix well. Press the crust into the bottom of the prepared pan.

Sprinkle the chocolate chips over the crust, then the pecans, then the coconut. Pour the caramel cream over the top. Bake for 25–30 minutes, until the edges are golden. Let cool before cutting into bars and serving.

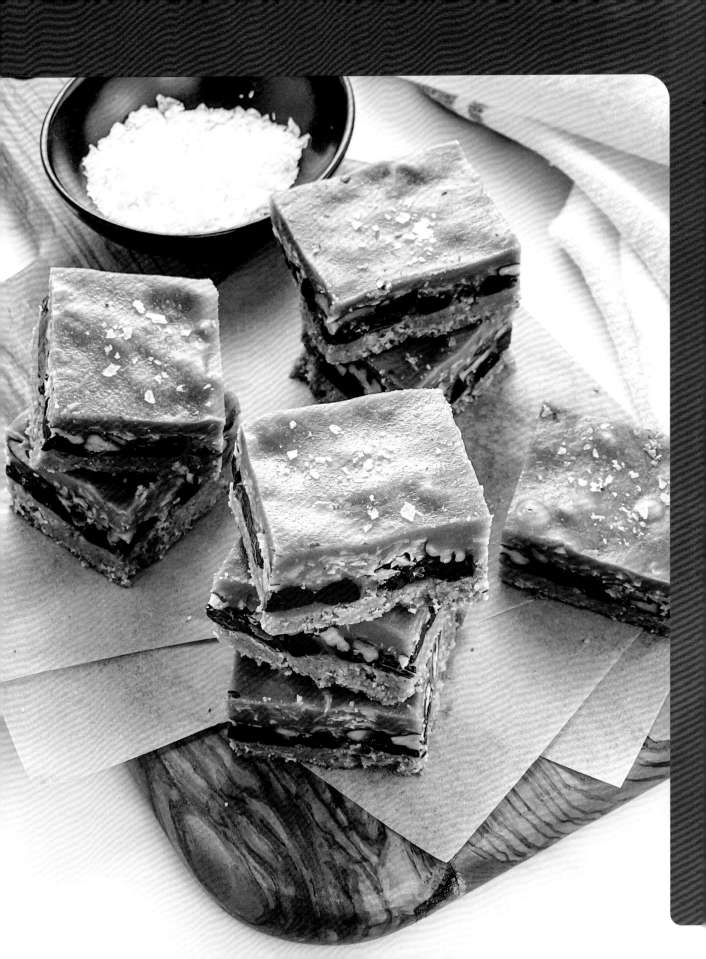

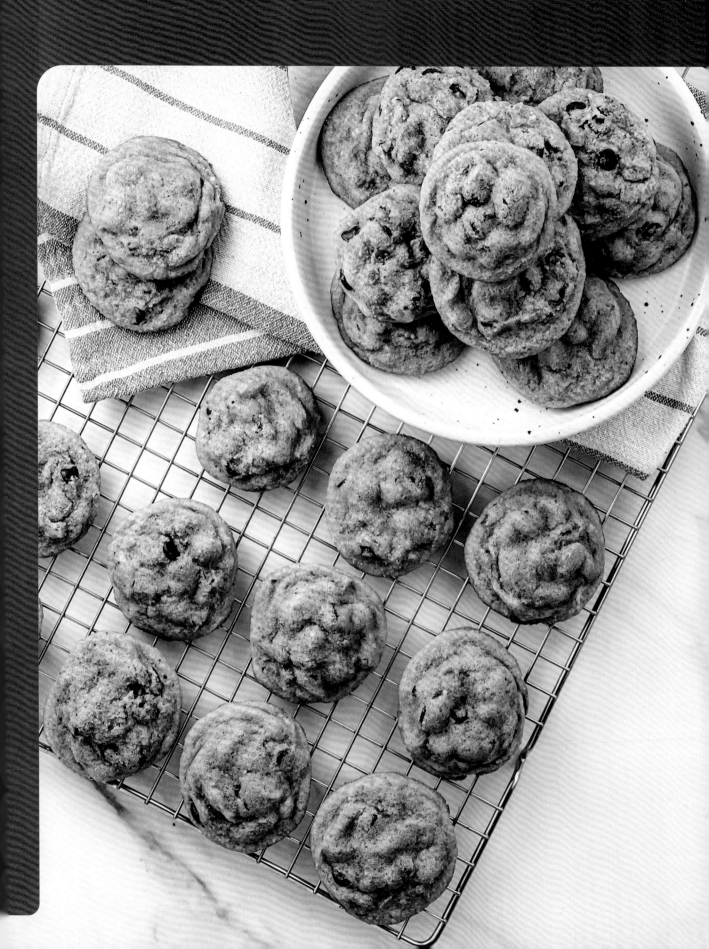

Chewy Chocolate Chip Cookies Ⓡ Ⓟ Ⓜ

Per cookie: Calories: 139 Fat: 12g Net Carb: 4g (11%) Protein: 3g
Makes 24 cookies | Prep time: 10 minutes | Bake time: 10 minutes

Preheat the oven to 350 degrees F. Line a rimmed baking sheet with parchment paper.

In the bowl of an electric mixer, beat the butter on high for 30 seconds. Add the Swerve, baking soda, and salt and beat on medium for 2 minutes, scraping down the sides as needed. Beat in the egg and vanilla. Beat in the almond flour. Stir in the chocolate pieces and pecans.

Drop heaping tablespoons of dough 2 inches apart on the prepared baking sheet. Sprinkle the tops with flaky sea salt. Bake for 8–10 minutes, until the edges are lightly browned. Transfer the parchment paper to a wire rack to cool.

8 tablespoons (1 stick) unsalted butter, room temperature
⅔ cup brown Swerve
½ teaspoon baking soda
½ teaspoon salt
1 large egg
1 tablespoon vanilla extract
2 cups almond flour
1 cup stevia-sweetened chocolate chips (such as Lily's)
½ cup pecans, chopped
Flaky sea salt, for sprinkling

Sweet and Salty Dessert Bark 🅡 🅟 🅜

Per serving: Calories: 253 Fat: 23g Net Carb: 5g (8%) Protein: 4g

Makes 8 servings | Prep time: 10 minutes, plus 20 minutes chilling time | Cook time: 5 minutes

1 cup coconut butter

½ cup unsweetened cocoa
   powder

1 teaspoon vanilla extract

⅓ cup confectioners Swerve,
   plus more to taste

½ teaspoon flaky sea salt

1 tablespoon pepitas

1 tablespoon chopped raw
   almonds

1 tablespoon shelled
   pistachios

Line a rimmed baking sheet with parchment paper.

Pour about an inch of water into a small saucepan and bring to a simmer. Put the coconut butter in a heatproof bowl and set it on top of the saucepan, making sure the bottom of the bowl does not touch the water below. Stir until melted and smooth. Remove the bowl from the heat and stir in the cocoa powder, vanilla, and Swerve.

Spread the melted chocolate mixture over the parchment paper on the baking sheet. Sprinkle with the flaky salt, pepitas, almonds, and pistachios. Chill until it hardens, about 20 minutes, then break the bark into pieces. Store in an airtight container in the refrigerator or freezer.

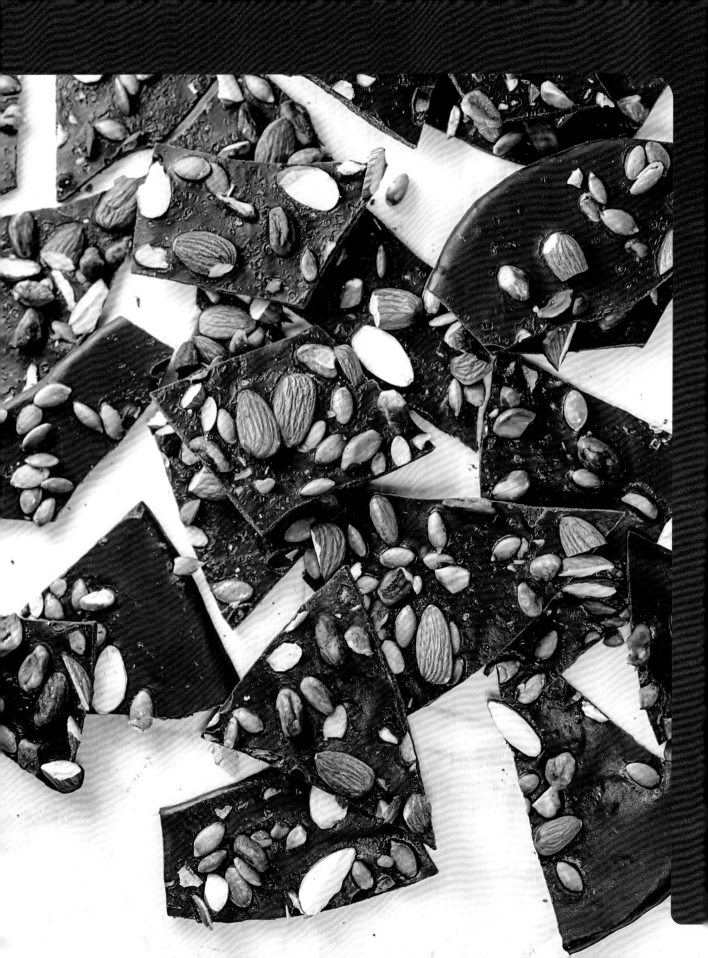

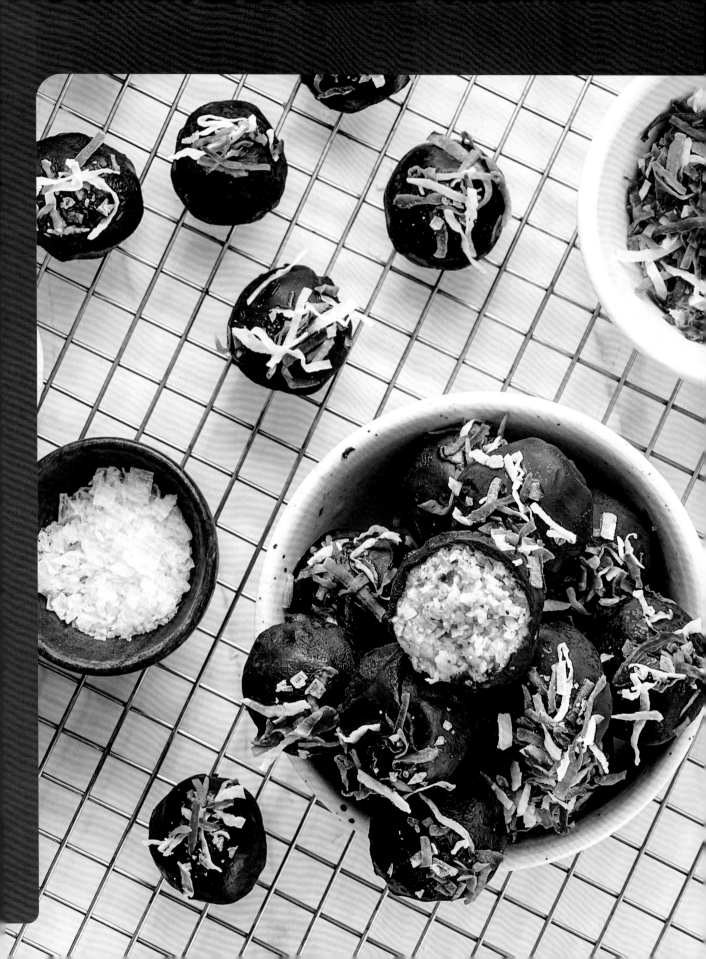

Chocolate Coconut Cream Truffles Ⓡ Ⓟ Ⓜ

Per truffle: Calories: 196 Fat: 19g Net Carb: 2g (5%) Protein: 2g
Makes 24 truffles | Prep time: 30 minutes | Bake time: 50 minutes

Preheat the oven to 350 degrees F. Line a rimmed baking sheet with parchment paper.

To make the topping, spread ½ cup of shredded coconut on the prepared baking sheet and roast, stirring every 3 minutes, until golden, about 9 minutes total. Remove from the oven and set aside.

To make the caramel cream, combine the cream, butter, and Swerve in a medium skillet and bring to a boil over medium heat, stirring often. Turn the heat down to low and simmer, stirring occasionally, until thick and creamy and reduced to ½ cup, about 20 minutes. Set aside to cool completely.

To make the filling, pulse the coconut in a food processor until fine. Add the caramel cream, melted butter, vanilla and coconut extracts, and confectioners Swerve. Pulse until fully combined. Cover and refrigerate for 20 minutes.

To make the chocolate, pour about an inch of water into a small saucepan and bring to a simmer. Put the coconut butter in a heatproof bowl and set it on top of the saucepan, making sure the bottom of the bowl does not touch the water below. Stir until melted and smooth. Remove the bowl from the heat and stir in the cocoa powder, vanilla, confectioners Swerve, and coconut oil.

Place a wire rack over the baking sheet. Form 24 balls with the coconut filling, about 1½ tablespoons each, and place on the rack. Spoon the melted chocolate over the truffles. Sprinkle with the toasted coconut and flaky salt. Chill until the chocolate sets, about 20 minutes.

Topping
½ cup unsweetened shredded coconut
Flaky sea salt

Caramel Cream
⅔ cup heavy cream
1 tablespoon unsalted butter
¼ cup brown Swerve

Filling
8 ounces unsweetened shredded coconut (about 4 cups)
2 tablespoons unsalted butter, melted
½ teaspoon vanilla extract
½ teaspoon coconut extract
3 tablespoons confectioners Swerve

Chocolate
1 cup coconut butter
½ cup unsweetened cocoa powder
1 teaspoon vanilla extract
⅓ cup confectioners Swerve
3 tablespoons coconut oil

Appendix: Expanded Food Lists

Here is a fuller list of smart foods to help control insulin, divided by food category (thanks to www.ruled.me and Insulin IQ for the resources):

Insulin-Friendly Choices—eat these until you're satiated.

Fats & Oils

Avocado oil

Coconut oil

Extra-virgin olive oil

Fish oil

Ghee

Lard or rendered animal fat

MCT oil

Dairy (limit your intake if you have sensitivities)

Butter

Cottage cheese

Cream cheese

Cheese (unprocessed)

Greek yogurt (full fat)

Heavy cream

Protein

All meats (beef, lamb, game)—choose grass-fed if you can

All poultry (chicken, turkey, and others)—choose pastured if you can

Eggs—choose pastured and eat the yolks

Fish and seafood—choose wild-caught and avoid farmed fish

Tofu and tempeh—if you are vegetarian or vegan

Vegetables & Fruits (aim for vegetables that grow aboveground)

Artichoke hearts

Asparagus

Avocados

Bamboo shoots

Bok choy

Celery

Cucumber

Green leafy vegetables (arugula, chard, lettuce, spinach, etc.)

Jicama

Leeks

Lemons

Limes

Mushrooms

Olives

Onions

Peppers (bell peppers, jalapeños, etc.)

Radishes

Watermelon

All herbs and spices (basil, cilantro, parsley, rosemary, thyme, etc.)

Fermented Foods

Apple cider vinegar

Kimchi

Pickles

Sauerkraut

Sourdough bread (look for real sourdough starter in ingredients)

Beverages

Coffee—black or with cream

Kombucha

Sparkling water—add lemon, lime, or apple cider vinegar

Tea

Unsweetened nut and seed milks (almond, coconut)

Condiments & Sweeteners

Mayonnaise (full fat)

Noncaloric sweeteners (erythritol, stevia, monk fruit, xylitol)

Salad dressings without sugar

Limit to 2 or fewer servings a day

Nuts, Seeds & Legumes

Almond flour and coconut flour

Almonds

Flaxseeds

Hazelnuts

Macadamia nuts

Nut butters

Peanuts

Pecans

Pine nuts

Pumpkin seeds

Sunflower seeds

Walnuts

Protein

Bacon with no added preservatives or starches

Fermented soy products

Powdered protein supplements

Vegetables, Fruit & Grains

Bean sprouts

Berries (blackberries, blueberries, cranberries, raspberries, strawberries)

Broccoli

Brussels sprouts

Cabbage

Cauliflower

Edamame

Eggplant

Kale

Okra

Snap peas

Barley pearls

Beverages

Alcoholic beverages (dry wines, clear alcohols, low-carb beer like Michelob Ultra and Select 55)

Flavored fruit drinks with noncaloric sweeteners (Bai, Zevia)

Whole milk

Condiments & Sweeteners

Greek yogurt dips

Hummus

Salad dressings containing 2 or fewer carbs or starches

Sugar alcohol sweeteners (malitol, sorbitol)

Avoid when possible or eat less than daily

Fats & Oils

Canola oil

Margarine

Peanut oil

Soybean oil

Trans fats

Dairy (avoid low-fat)

Condensed milk

High-sugar ice creams

Skim or low-fat milk

Protein: avoid any proteins that are breaded or served with sugary sauces

Vegetables, Fruits & Grains

Apples

Apricots

Bananas

Canned fruits

Cherries

Dates

Grapefruit

Grapes

Jam, jelly, and preserves

Mango

Melons

Oranges

Peaches

Pears

Plantains

Raisins

Beverages

Fruit juice

Soda, including diet soda

Sports drinks (Gatorade)

Alcohol (most beer, sweet wines, mixers, and cocktails)

Condiments & Sweeteners

Agave

Aspartame

Corn syrup and high-fructose corn syrup

Fructose

Honey

Maple syrup

Sucralose

Sugar (white and brown)

Acknowledgments

Benjamin Bikman

My wife and children continue to be my greatest source of motivation and support. Being the husband and father of my family will forever be my greatest accomplishment.

This book would not have happened if it weren't for the encouragement of Glenn Yeffeth, whose enthusiasm for *Why We Get Sick* prompted a companion book. Thankfully, when I shared with Glenn my general lack of skill at meal and exercise planning, we were able to convince Diana Keuilian to come aboard. By having her be the expert on "what to do," I was able to focus solely on "what to know" (a comfortable space for a professor). And, of course, my agent, Faye Atchison, continues to be my greatest cheerleader—she was the first to believe my ideas had value.

As before, my editor, Claire Schulz, was essential in ordering the chaos of writing a book. If Glenn planted the seed of this book, Claire ensured it was cared for and harvested. To her and all the staff at BenBella, thank you once again for helping a professor take ideas from the classroom to the world.

Diana Keuilian

I am deeply grateful to Glenn Yeffeth for introducing me to Dr. Ben Bikman and creating the opportunity for this exciting collaboration. As a reader and enthusiast of *Why We Get Sick*, it is an incredible honor to be part of this companion book.

My husband, Bedros, taught me how to lift weights some twenty years ago, and he continues to inspire me in the gym and in life. All the credit for the shred burn workout goes to you, my love.

My children, Andrew and Chloe, tasted all of the recipe creations in this book and provided me with their honest feedback. Thank you for being my favorite taste testers.

Many thanks to Claire Schulz for her beautiful work in editing this book, and to all the amazing staff at BenBella for their support.

Notes

Introduction

1   Walton, C. M., et al. *Improvement in glycemic and lipid profiles in type 2 diabetics with a 90-day ketogenic diet.* J Diabetes Res, 2019. 2019(8681959): p. 1-6.

2   de la Monte, S. M., and J. R. Wands. *Alzheimer's disease is type 3 diabetes-evidence reviewed.* J Diabetes Sci Technol, 2008. **2**(6): p. 1101-3.

3   Reaven, G. M. *Relationship between insulin resistance and hypertension.* Diabetes Care, 1991. **14 Suppl 4**: 33-8.

4   Kraft, J. R. *Hyperinsulinemia: the common denominator of subjective idiopathic tinnitus and other idiopathic central and peripheral neurootologic disorders.* Int Tinnitus J, 1995. **1**(1): p. 46-53.

5   Wang, H. S., and T. H. Wang. *Polycystic ovary syndrome (PCOS), insulin resistance and insulin-like growth factors (IGfs)/IGF-binding proteins (IGFBPs).* Chang Gung Med J, 2003. 26(8): p. 540-53; Yao, F., et al. *Erectile dysfunction may be the first clinical sign of insulin resistance and endothelial dysfunction in young men.* Clin Res Cardiol, 2013. **102**(9): p. 645-51.

Chapter 1

1   Araujo, J., J. Cai, and J. Stevens. *Prevalence of optimal metabolic health in American adults: National Health and Nutrition Examination Survey 2009-2016.* Metab Syndr Relat Disord, 2019. **17**(1): p. 46-52.

2   Godsland, I. F., C. Walton, and V. Wynn. *Role of glucose and insulin resistance in development of type 2 diabetes mellitus.* Lancet, 1992. **340**(9): p. 1347-8.

3   Hjermann, I. *The metabolic cardiovascular syndrome: syndrome X, Reaven's syndrome, insulin resistance syndrome, atherothrombogenic syndrome.* J Cardiovasc Pharmacol, 1992. **20 Suppl 8**: p. S5-10.

4   Araujo, J., J. Cai, and J. Stevens. *Prevalence of optimal metabolic health in American adults: National Health and Nutrition Examination Survey 2009-2016.* Metab Syndr Relat Disord, 2019. **17**(1): p. 46-52.

5   Johnson, J. L., et al. *Identifying prediabetes using fasting insulin levels.* Endocr Pract, 2010. **16**(1): p. 47-52.

6   Crofts, C., et al. *Identifying hyperinsulinaemia in the absence of impaired glucose tolerance: an examination of the Kraft database.* Diabetes Res Clinic Pract, 2016. **118**: p. 50-57.

7   Guerrero-Romero, F., et al. *The product of triglycerides and glucose, a simple measure of insulin sensitivity. Comparison with the euglycemic-hyperinsulinemic clamp.* J Clinic Endocrinol Metab, 2010. **95**(7): p. 3347-51.

8   Young, K. A., et al. *The triglyceride to high-density lipoprotein cholesterol (TG/HDL-C) ratio as a predictor of insulin resistance, beta-cell function, and diabetes in Hispanics and African Americans.* J Diabetes Complications, 2019. **33**(2): p. 118-22; Giannini, C., et al. *The triglyceride-to-HDL cholesterol ratio: association with insulin resistance in obese youths of different ethnic backgrounds.* Diabetes Care, 2011. **34**(8): p. 1869-74.

9   Spalding, K. L., et al. *Dynamics of fat cell turnover in humans.* Nature, 2008. **453**(7196): p. 783-7.

10 Pandi-Perumal, et al. *Melatonin and sleep in aging population.* Exp Gerontol, 2005. **40**(12): p. 911-25.

11   Van Cauter, E. *Sleep disturbances and insulin resistance.* Diabet Med, 2011. **28**(12): p. 1455-62.

12   Willey, K. A., and M. A. Singh. *Battling insulin resistance in elderly obese people with type 2 diabetes: bring on the heavy weights.* Diabetes Care, 2003. **26**(5): p. 1580-88.

Chapter 2

1   Furmli, S., et al. *Therapeutic use of intermittent fasting for people with type 2 diabetes as an alternative to insulin.* BMJ Case Rep, 2018. **2018**.

2   Horne, B. D., et al. *Relation of routine, periodic fasting to risk of diabetes mellitus, and coronary artery disease in patients undergoing coronary angiography.* Am J Cardiol, 2012. **109**(11): p. 1558-62.

3   Hutchison, A. T., and L. K. Heilbronn. *Metabolic impacts of altering meal frequency and timing—Does when we eat matter?* Biochimie, 2016. **124**: p. 187-97; Kahleova, H., et al. *Eating two larger meals a day (breakfast and lunch) is more effective than six smaller meals in a reduced-energy regimen for patients with type 2 diabetes: a randomised crossover study.* Diabetologia, 2014. **57**(8): p. 1552-60.

4   Ravussin, E., et al. *Early time-restricted feeding reduces appetite and increases fat oxidation but does not affect energy expenditure in humans.* Obesity (Silver Spring), 2019. **27**(8): p. 1244-54.

5   Bolli, G. B., et al. *Demonstration of a dawn phenomenon in normal human volunteers.* Diabetes, 1984. **33**(12): p. 1150-3.

6   Jarrett, R. J., et al. *Diurnal variation in oral glucose tolerance: blood sugar and plasma insulin levels morning, afternoon, and evening.* Br Med J, 1972. **1**(5794): p. 199-201.

7   Dimitrov, S., et al. *Cortisol and epinephrine control opposing circadian rhythms in T cell subsets.* Blood, 2009. **113**(21): p. 5134-43.

8   Schmidt, M. I., et al. *The dawn phenomenon, an early morning glucose rise: implications for diabetic intraday blood glucose variation.* Diabetes Care, 1981. **4**(6): p. 579-85.

9   Carrasco-Benso, M. P., et al. *Human adipose tissue expresses intrinsic circadian rhythm in insulin sensitivity.* FASEB J, 2016. **30**(9): p. 311723.

10   Chakrabarti, P., et al. *Insulin inhibits lipolysis in adipocytes via the evolutionarily conserved mTORC1-Egr1-ATGL-mediated pathway.* Mol Cell Biol, 2013. **33**(18): p. 3659-66.

11   Stahl, A., et al. *Insulin causes fatty acid transport protein translocation and enhanced fatty acid uptake in adipocytes.* Dev Cell, 2002. **2**(4): p. 477-88.

12   Zakaria, A. *Ramadan-like fasting reduces carbonyl stress and improves glycemic control in insulin treated type 2 diabetes mellitus patients.* Life Sci, 2013. **10**(9): p. 384-90.

13   Mehanna, H. M., J. Moledina, and J. Travis. *Refeeding syndrome: what it is, and how to prevent and treat it.* BMJ, 2008. **336**(7659): p. 1495-8.

14   Silva, A. S., et al. *Treatment of morbid obesity with adjustable gastric band: preliminary report.* Obes Surg, 1999. **9**(2): p. 194-7.

15   Heilbronn, L. K., et al. *Glucose tolerance and skeletal muscle gene expression in response to alternate day fasting.* Obes Res, 2005. **13**(3): p. 574-81.

16   Harvie, M. N., et al. *The effects of intermittent or continuous energy restriction on weight loss and metabolic disease risk markers: a randomized trial in young overweight women.* Int J Obes (Lond), 2011. **35**(5): p. 714-27.

17   Harvie, M., et al. *The effect of intermittent energy and carbohydrate restriction v. daily energy restriction on weight loss and metabolic disease risk markers in overweight women.* British J Nutr, 2013. **110**(8): p. 1534-47.

18   Chiofalo, B., et al. *Fasting as possible complementary approach for polycystic ovary syndrome: Hope or hype?* Med hypotheses, 2017. **105**: p. 1-3.

Fasting and Sleep (sidebar on page 31)

1   Lack, L. C., et al. *The relationship between insomnia and body temperatures.* Sleep Med Rev, 2008. **12**(4): p. 307-17.

2   Kenny, G. P., R. J. Sigal, and R. McGinn. *Body temperature regulation in diabetes.* Temperature (Austin), 2016. **3**(1): p. 119-45.

3   Kenny, G. P., et al. *Older adults with type 2 diabetes store more heat during exercise.* Med Sci Sports Exerc, 2013. **45**(10): p. 1906-14.

4   Green, J. H., and I. A. Macdonald. *The influence of intravenous glucose on body temperature.* Q J Exp Physiol, 1981. **66**(4): p. 465-73; Welle, S., and R. G. Campbell. *Stimulation of thermogenesis by carbohydrate overfeeding. Evidence against sympathetic nervous system mediation.* J Clin Invest, 1983. **71**(4): p. 916-25.

5   Jalilolghadr, S., et al. *Effect of low and high glycaemic index drink on sleep pattern in children.* J Pak Med Assoc, 2011. **61**(6): p. 533-36.

Chapter 3

1   Traylor, D. A., S. H. M. Gorissen, and S. M. Phillips. *Perspective: protein requirements and optimal intakes in aging: Are we ready to recommend more than the recommended daily allowance?* Adv Nutr, 2018. **9**(3): p. 171-82.

2   Buckman, M. T., et al. *Effect of fasting on alanine-stimulated insulin and glucagon secretion.* Metabolism, 1973. **22**(10): p. 1253-62.

3   Volek, J. S., et al. *Carbohydrate restriction has a more favorable impact on the metabolic syndrome than a low fat diet.* Lipids, 2009. **44**(4): p. 297-309.

4   Pellinen, T., et al. *Replacing dietary animal-source proteins with plant-source proteins changes dietary intake and status of vitamins and minerals in healthy adults: a 12-week randomized controlled trial.* Eur J Nutr, 2022. **61**(3): p. 1391-404.

5   Linderoth, A., et al. *Binding and the effect of the red kidney bean lectin, phytohaemagglutinin, in the gastrointestinal tract of suckling rats.* Br J Nutr, 2006. **95**(1): p. 105-15.

6   Fredlund, K., et al. *Absorption of zinc and retention of calcium: dose-dependent inhibition by phytate.* J Trace Elem Med Biol, 2006. **20**(1): p. 49-57.

7   Delimont, N. M., M. D. Haub, and B. L. Lindshield. *The impact of tannin consumption on iron bioavailability and status: a narrative review.* Curr Dev Nutr, 2017. **1**(2): p. 1-12.

8   Clean Label Project. *New study of protein powders from Clean Label Project finds elevated levels of heavy metals and BPA in 53 leading brands.* February 27, 2018. https://cleanlabelproject.org/blog-post/new-study-of-protein-powders-from-clean-label-project-finds-elevated-levels-of-heavy-metals-and-bpa-in-53-leading-brands/.

9   Mukherjee, R., R. Chakraborty, and A. Dutta. *Role of fermentation in improving nutritional quality of soybean meal-a review.* Asian-Australas J Anim Sci, 2016. **29**(11): p. 1523-9.

10   Kiczorowski, P., et al. *Effect of fermentation of chosen vegetables on the nutrient, mineral, and biocomponent profile in human and animal nutrition.* Sci Rep, 2022. **12**(1): p. 13422.

11   Gass, J., et al. *Enhancement of dietary protein digestion by conjugated bile acids.* Gastroenterology, 2007. **133**(1): p. 16-23.

12   van Vliet, S., et al. *Consumption of whole eggs promotes greater stimulation of postexercise muscle protein synthesis than consumption of isonitrogenous amounts of egg whites in young men.* Am J Clin Nutr, 2017. **106**(6): p. 1401-12.

Chapter 4

1   Ramsden, C. E., et al. *Re-evaluation of the traditional diet-heart hypothesis: analysis of recovered data from Minnesota Coronary Experiment (1968-73).* BMJ, 2016. **353**: p. i1246.

2   Forsythe, C. E., et al. *Comparison of low fat and low carbohydrate diets on circulating fatty acid composition and markers of inflammation.* Lipids, 2008. **43**(1): p. 65-77.

3   Kokatnur, M. G., et al. *Fatty acid composition of human adipose tissue from two anatomical sites in a biracial community.* Am J Clin Nutr, 1979. **32**(11): p. 2198-205.

4   Chiu, S., et al. *Comparison of the DASH (Dietary Approaches to Stop Hypertension) diet and a higher-fat DASH diet on blood pressure and lipids and lipoproteins: a randomized controlled trial.* Am J Clin Nutr, 2016. **103**(2): p. 341-7.

5   Fageras Bottcher, M., et al. *A TLR4 polymorphism is associated with asthma and reduced lipopolysaccharide-induced interleukin-12(p70) responses in Swedish children.* J Allergy Clin Immunol, 2004. **114**(3): p. 561-7.

6   Shor, R., et al. *Low serum LDL cholesterol levels and the risk of fever, sepsis, and malignancy.* Ann Clin Lab Sci, 2007. **37**(4): p. 343-8; Kaysen, G. A., et al. *Lipid levels are inversely associated with infectious and all-cause mortality: international MONDO study results.* J Lipid Res, 2018. **59**(8): p. 1519-28.

7   Liu, Y., et al. *Association between low density lipoprotein cholesterol and all-cause mortality: results from the NHANES 1999-2014.* Sci Rep, 2021. **11**(1): p. 22111; Schatz, I. J., et al. *Cholesterol and all-cause mortality in elderly people from the Honolulu Heart Program: a cohort study.* Lancet, 2001. **358**(9279): p. 351-5; Wu, W., et al. *Low and high-density lipoprotein cholesterol and 10-year mortality in community-dwelling older adults: the Shanghai Aging Study.* Front Med (Lausanne), 2022. **9**: p. 783618.

8   Tan, L. C., et al. *Dietary cholesterol, fats and risk of Parkinson's disease in the Singapore Chinese Health Study.* J Neurol Neurosurg Psychiatry, 2016. **87**(1): p. 86-92.

9   Hamalainen, E. K., et al. *Decrease of serum total and free testosterone during a low-fat high-fibre diet.* J Steroid Biochem, 1983. **18**(3): p. 369-70.

10   Berghoff, S. A., et al. *Dietary cholesterol promotes repair of demyelinated lesions in the adult brain.* Nat Commun, 2017. **8**: p. 14241.

11   Luczaj, W., and E. Skrzydlewska. *DNA damage caused by lipid peroxidation products.* Cell Mol Biol Lett, 2003. **8**(2): p. 391-413.

12   Ramsden, C. E., et al. *Re-evaluation of the traditional diet-heart hypothesis: analysis of recovered data from Minnesota Coronary Experiment (1968-73).* BMJ, 2016. **353**: p. i1246.

13   Ramsden, C. E., et al. *Use of dietary linoleic acid for secondary prevention of coronary heart disease and death: evaluation of recovered data from the Sydney Diet Heart Study and updated meta-analysis.* BMJ, 2013. **346**: p. e8707.

14   Guyenet, S. J., and S. E. Carlson. *Increase in adipose tissue linoleic acid of US adults in the last half century.* Adv Nutr, 2015. **6**(6): p. 660-4.

15   Budowski, P. *The omega-3 fatty acid peroxidation paradox.* Redox Rep, 1996. **2**(1): p. 75-77.

16   Smith, G. I., et al. *Dietary omega-3 fatty acid supplementation increases the rate of muscle protein synthesis in older adults: a randomized controlled trial.* American J Clin Nutr, 2011. **93**(2): p. 402-12.

17   Leiria, L. O., et al. *12-Lipoxygenase regulates cold adaptation and glucose metabolism by producing the omega-3 lipid 12-HEPE from brown fat.* Cell Metab, 2019. **30**(4): p. 768-83.e7.

Chapter 5

1   Sjostrom, L. *Fatty acid synthesis de novo in adipose tissue from obese subjects on a hypercaloric high-carbohydrate diet.* Scand J Clin Lab Invest, 1973. **32**(4): p. 339-49.

2   American Diabetes Association. *5. Facilitating behavior change and well-being to improve health outcomes: standards of medical care in diabetes-2021.* Diabetes Care, 2021. **44 Suppl 1**: p. S53-72.

3   Hu, T., et al. *Effects of low-carbohydrate diets versus low-fat diets on metabolic risk factors: a meta-analysis of randomized controlled clinical trials.* Am J Epidemiol, 2012. **176 Suppl 7**:

p. S44-54; Santos, F. L., et al. *Systematic review and meta-analysis of clinical trials of the effects of low carbohydrate diets on cardiovascular risk factors.* Obes Rev, 2012. **13**(11): p. 1048-66.

4   Institute of Medicine of the National Academies. *Dietary Reference Intakes for Energy, Carbohydrate, Fiber, Fat, Fatty Acids, Cholesterol, Protein, and Amino Acids,* chapter 1. Washington, DC: National Academies Press, 2002/2005. https://nap.nationalacademies.org/read/10490/chapter/1.

5   Yan, L., et al. *Effects of the physical form of the diet on food intake, growth, and body composition changes in mice.* J Am Assoc Lab Anim Sci, 2011. **50**(4): p. 488-94.

6   Demirkesen-Bicak, H., et al. *Effect of different fermentation condition on estimated glycemic index, in vitro starch digestibility, and textural and sensory properties of sourdough bread.* Foods, 2021. **10**(3): p. 514.

7   Najjar, N., N. Adra, and N. Hwalla. *Glycemic and insulinemic responses to hot vs cooled potato in males with varied insulin sensitivity.* Nutr Res, 2004. **24**(12): p. 993-1004.

8   Adapted from Ruled.me.

9   Patil, J. *Processed Carbohydrates Are Addictive, Brain Study Suggests.* Western Kentucky University, 2013. https://www.wku.edu/news/articles/index.php?view=article&articleid=2332.

10   Shukla, A. P., et al. *The impact of food order on postprandial glycaemic excursions in prediabetes.* Diabetes Obes Metab, 2019. **21**(2): p. 377-81.

11   Taylor, H. L., et al. *Post-exercise carbohydrate-energy replacement attenuates insulin sensitivity and glucose tolerance the following morning in healthy adults.* Nutrients, 2018. **10**(2): p. 123.

12   Estafanos, S., et al. *Carbohydrate-energy replacement following high-intensity interval exercise blunts next-day glycemic control in untrained women.* Front Nutr, 2022. **9**: p. 868511.

13   Walsh, C. O., et al. *Effects of diet composition on postprandial energy availability during weight loss maintenance.* PloS One, 2013. **8**(3): p. e58172.

14   Ebbeling, C. B., et al. *Effects of dietary composition on energy expenditure during weight-loss maintenance.* JAMA, 2012. **307**(24): p. 2627-34.

Uric Acid and Inflammation (sidebar on page 52)

1   Wan, X., et al. *Uric acid regulates hepatic steatosis and insulin resistance through the NLRP3 inflammasome-dependent mechanism.* J Hepatol, 2016. **64**(4): p. 925-32.

Ben's Favorite Fermented Food (sidebar on page 53)

1   Hu, J., et al. *Short-chain fatty acid acetate stimulates adipogenesis and mitochondrial biogenesis via GPR43 in brown adipocytes.* Endocrinology, 2016. **157**(5): p. 1881-94.

2   Johnston, C. S., C. M. Kim, and A. J. Buller. *Vinegar improves insulin sensitivity to a high-carbohydrate meal in subjects with insulin resistance or type 2 diabetes.* Diabetes Care, 2004. **27**(1): p. 281-2; Liatis, S., et al. *Vinegar reduces postprandial hyperglycaemia in patients with type II diabetes when added to a high, but not to a low, glycaemic index meal.* Eur J Clin Nutr, 2010. **64**(7): p. 727-32; Johnston, C. S., A. M. White, and S. M. Kent. *Preliminary evidence that regular vinegar ingestion favorably influences hemoglobin A1c values in individuals with type 2 diabetes mellitus.* Diabetes Res Clin Pract, 2009. **84**(2): p. e15-17.

3   White, A. M., and C. S. Johnston. *Vinegar ingestion at bedtime moderates waking glucose concentrations in adults with well-controlled type 2 diabetes.* Diabetes Care, 2007. **30**(11): p. 2814-5.

Hydrate, Hydrate! (sidebar on page 57)

1   Stookey, J. D., et al. *Underhydration is associated with obesity, chronic diseases, and death within 3 to 6 years in the U.S. population aged 51-70 years.* Nutrients, 2020. **12**(4): p. 905.

2   Keller, U., et al. *Effects of changes in hydration on protein, glucose and lipid metabolism in man: impact on health.* Eur J Clin Nutr, 2003. **57 Suppl 2**: p. S69-74.

What About Alcohol? (sidebar on page 59)

1   Wilson, D. F., and F. M. Matschinsky. *Ethanol metabolism: The good, the bad, and the ugly.* Medical Hypotheses, 2020. 140: p. 109638.

2   Liu, J. *Ethanol and liver: Recent insights into the mechanisms of ethanol-induced fatty liver.* World J. Gastroenterol, 2014. **20**(40): p. 14672–85.

3   Ibid.

4   Rehm, J., et al. *Global burden of alcoholic liver diseases.* J Hepatol, 2013. **59**(1): p. 160-8.

5   Byrne, C. D. *Ectopic fat, insulin resistance and non-alcoholic fatty liver disease.* Proceedings of the Nutrition Society, 2013. **72**(4): p. 412-9.

Chapter 6

1   Ferguson, M. A., et al. *Effects of exercise training and its cessation on components of the insulin resistance syndrome in obese children.* Int J Obes Relat Metab Disord, 1999. **23**(8): p. 889-95; Miller, J. P., et al. *Strength training increases insulin action in healthy 50- to 65-yr-old men.* J Appl Physiol (1985), 1994. **77**(3): p. 1122-7.

2   Lehmann, R., et al. *Loss of abdominal fat and improvement of the cardiovascular risk profile by regular moderate exercise training in patients with NIDDM.* Diabetologia, 1995. **38**, p. 1313-1319.

3   Hughes, V. A., et al. *Exercise increases muscle GLUT-4 levels and insulin action in subjects with impaired glucose tolerance.* The American Journal of Physiology, 1993. **264**: p. E855-862.

4   Dunstan, D. W., et al. *Breaking up prolonged sitting reduces postprandial glucose and insulin responses.* Diabetes Care, 2012. **35**(5): p. 976-83.

5   Hamburg, N. M., et al. *Physical inactivity rapidly induces insulin resistance and microvascular dysfunction in healthy volunteers.* Arterioscler Thromb Vasc Biol, 2007. **27**(12): p. 2650-6.

6   Pereira, A. F., et al. *Muscle tissue changes with aging.* Acta Med Port, 2013. **26**(1): p. 51-5.

7   Tabata, I., et al. *Resistance training affects GLUT-4 content in skeletal muscle of humans after 19 days of head-down bed rest.* J Appl Physiol (1985), 1999. **86**(3): p. 909-14.

8   Eriksson, J., et al. *Aerobic endurance exercise or circuit-type resistance training for individuals with impaired glucose tolerance?* Horm Metab Res, 1998. **30**(1): p. 37-41.

9   Lee, S., et al. *Effects of aerobic versus resistance exercise without caloric restriction on abdominal fat, intrahepatic lipid, and insulin sensitivity in obese adolescent boys: a randomized, controlled trial.* Diabetes, 2012. **61**(11): p. 2787-95.

10   Yardley, J. E., et al. *Resistance versus aerobic exercise: acute effects on glycemia in type 1 diabetes.* Diabetes Care, 2013. **36**(3): p. 537-42.

11   Grontved, A., et al. *A prospective study of weight training and risk of type 2 diabetes mellitus in men.* Archives of Internal Medicine, 2012. **172**: 1306-12.

12   Kavookjian, J., B. M. Elswick, and T. Whetsel. *Interventions for being active among individuals with diabetes: a systematic review of the literature.* Diabetes Educ, 2007. **33**(6): p. 962-90.

13   Segerstrom, A. B., et al. *Impact of exercise intensity and duration on insulin sensitivity in women with T2D.* Eur J Intern Med, 2010. **21**(5): p. 404-8.

14   Babraj, J. A., et al. *Extremely short duration high intensity interval training substantially improves insulin action in young healthy males.* BMC Endocr Disord, 2009. **9**: p. 3

15   Ismail, A. D., et al. *The effect of short duration resistance training on insulin sensitivity and muscle adaptations in overweight men.* Exp Physiol, 2019. **104**(4): p. 540-5.

16   Mancilla, R., et al. *Exercise training elicits superior metabolic effects when performed in the afternoon compared to morning in metabolically compromised humans.* Physiol Rep, 2021. **8**(24): p. e14669.

Post-exercise Cool Down/Warm Up (sidebar on page 68)

1   Hesketh, K., et al. *Passive heat therapy in sedentary humans increases skeletal muscle capillarization and eNOS content but not mitochondrial density or GLUT4 content.* Am J Physiol Heart Circ Physiol, 2019. **317**(1): p. H114-23.

Chapter 7

1   Spiegel, K., R. Leproult, and E. Van Cauter. *Impact of sleep debt on metabolic and endocrine function.* Lancet, 1999. **354**(9188): p. 1435-9.

2   Sweeney, E. L., et al. *Skeletal muscle insulin signaling and whole-body glucose metabolism following acute sleep restriction in healthy males.* Physiol Rep, 2017. **5**(23): p. e13498.

3   Petrowski, K., et al. *Increase in cortisol concentration due to standardized bright and blue light exposure on saliva cortisol in the morning following sleep laboratory.* Stress, 2021. **24**(3): p.331-7.

4   Faraut, B., et al. *Daytime exposure to blue-enriched light counters the effects of sleep restriction on cortisol, testosterone, alpha-amylase and executive processes.* Front Neurosci, 2019. **13**: p. 1366.

5   Jalilolghadr, S., et al. *Effect of low and high glycaemic index drink on sleep pattern in children.* J Pak Med Assoc, 2011. **61**(6): p. 533-6.

6   Ma, X., et al. *The effect of diaphragmatic breathing on attention, negative affect and stress in healthy adults.* Front Psychol, 2017. **8**: p. 874.

Index

About the Authors

Benjamin Bikman earned his PhD in bioenergetics and was a postdoctoral fellow with the Duke–National University of Singapore, studying metabolic disorders. Currently, his professional focus as a scientist and professor (Brigham Young University) is to better understand the origins and consequences of metabolic disorders, including obesity and diabetes, with a particular emphasis on the role of insulin. He frequently publishes his research in peer-reviewed journals and presents at international science and public meetings.

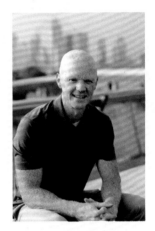

Photo by Leah Aldous

Diana Keuilian is passionate about creating wholesome versions of your favorite foods. She removes the gluten, soy, grains, and cane sugar from traditional comfort food recipes like cake, tacos, cookies, waffles, enchiladas, and more. This hobby propelled her to start the popular blog RealHealthyRecipes.com, where she shares hundreds of delicious recipes and mouthwatering photos. She lives in Southern California with her husband and two children.

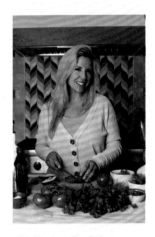

Photo by Anna Frenkel

Now that you know HOW NOT TO GET SICK, learn WHY WE GET SICK.

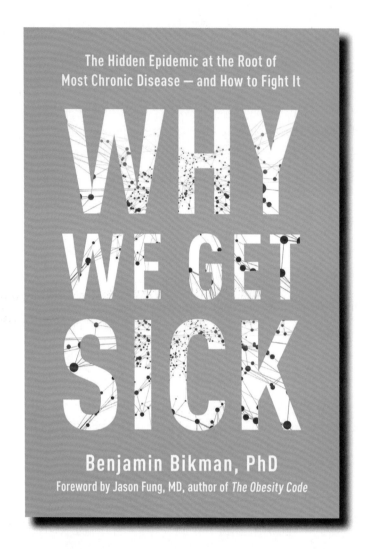

The Hidden Epidemic at the Root of Most Chronic Disease — and How to Fight It

WHY WE GET SICK

Benjamin Bikman, PhD

Foreword by Jason Fung, MD, author of *The Obesity Code*

Discover the groundbreaking research linking many diseases to one root cause: **insulin resistance**. In this companion book, you'll learn what it is, why it happens, and how it affects nearly every system in our bodies.

Available everywhere books are sold.